Advance Reviews

"Sandi makes the toughest journey seem refreshingly funny. Every doctor, comedian and patient should read this great book."
~ **Neil Leiberman**, The Comedy Coach®

"Love the raw honesty and humor. MS babe who got a stem cell transplant—that alone is a miracle."
~ **Christy Evans Jordan**, has MS

"I dog-earred over 20 pages that made me laugh out loud or burst in tears. I was awed by your journey, uplifted by your triumphs and overwhelmed by the simple message of family forever."
~ **Melissa Berger**

"Spell-binding—rings true on every level. Inspiring and empowering for anyone facing challenges they think are so insurmountable that they cannot be overcome."
~ **Lynn Ruth Miller**, author of *Starving Hearts*

"Sandi incorporates some great laughs into her MS story, proving that she's not only a funny comedian but a strong woman as well."
~ **Heather Barbieri**, owner of Rooster T. Feathers

"Wonderful, amazing, heartbreaking, inspiring."
~ **Britta Wilder**, writer and painter

"Inspiration for anyone diagnosed with a serious disease. It shows that IT IS possible to not only beat the odds, but to pursue your passion at the same time."

~ **John DeKoven**, Bunjo's Comedy Club

"Really good read. Thanks for the insightful look into your life. You're a brave woman."

~ **Rich Stimbra**, Asst. Dir. SFCC

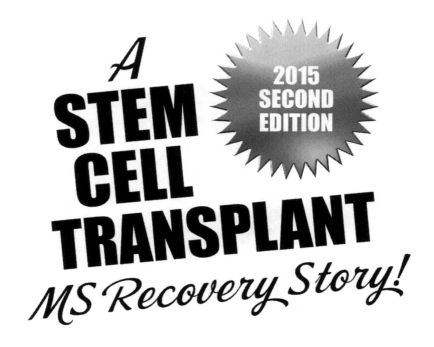

A STEM CELL TRANSPLANT

2015 SECOND EDITION

MS Recovery Story!

Beating Multiple Sclerosis with Humor, Hope & Science

Sandi Selvi

Keynote Speaker, Stand-up Comedian, Stem-Cell Recipient & MS Survivor

FORMERLY TITLED *WON'T DO STAND-UP IN A WHEELCHAIR*

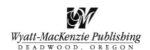

Wyatt-MacKenzie Publishing
DEADWOOD, OREGON

A Stem Cell Transplant MS Recovery Story:
Beating Multiple Sclerosis with Humor, Hope & Science

Previously titled
Won't Do Stand-Up in a Wheelchair
An M.S. Recovery Story

Sandi Selvi

S E C O N D   E D I T I O N

ISBN: 978-1-936214-10-5
Library of Congress Control Number: 2010923580

Author Photography by Sharon Hall Photography

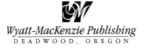

Wyatt-MacKenzie Publishing
D E A D W O O D ,   O R E G O N

15115 Highway 36, Deadwood, Oregon 97430
541-964-3314
www.wyattmackenzie.com

Dedication

I dedicate this book to my husband Rob, our two sons Jim and Tom, and my nephew (and third son) Garrett.
Thanks for carrying on with the tradition that family is always first.

Acknowledgments

I want to thank those people who made this book a reality.

Thanks from the bottom of my heart, Jodi, Katelyn, Pam, Beth, Helen, Suzie, Neil, Judy, Vic, my family, my doctors…and Scott.

Contents

Introduction

The day after my fortieth birthday, my lung was punctured during a medical procedure to place a port in my chest. This port had nothing to do with a class of very sweet wines, mostly dark red, originally from Portugal, which, by the way, was the only port I knew existed before the procedure. This port had two tubes that were surgically implanted under my clavicle, directly into an artery, to deliver I.V. solutions, blood, my own stem cells, and potassium (lots of potassium). The doctors said the port would make it easier to take out the blood samples they would need daily, and it would be a whole lot easier to put the things I would need back in me later. Only problem: the doctor just happened to, as he says, "nick" my right lung on the way in.

Even with the, as I call it, "lung puncture," I would do it all again. It's almost like I never had M.S. Sure, it had its side effects, but my M.S. is totally back to manageable now. I no longer tremble all the time. I still have muscle spasms, but not like before. Best of all, I no longer need my cane to walk. It's funny, I have no pictures of me with a cane. I used that thing for four years, and I can't even remember anyone ever taking a photo of me with it. I have hundreds of pictures of me modeling, at my wedding, with the kids, and on stage, but not one with a cane. I wonder if that is significant?

It seems like the Sandi I am now is so different from the one ten years ago. I sometimes read my own journal to remind myself of what I went through and how fortunate I am to be alive. I am fortunate to have been given a second chance at life. How many people can say that? So, you ask, what am I going to do now with my second chance? My favorite entry in my journal might be a hint. It reminds me how laughter is *indeed* the best medicine.

Thursday, March 16, 2000—15 Days to Transplant

We arrived at the hospital at 1 p.m. Checked in, then were put in a room. They told us the wait might be longer than we had anticipated and that I should just rest there until they called me. By 7 p.m., I was getting a little nervous. Finally the procedure began. At about 8 p.m., I was in recovery, feeling a little sore. I kept telling the nurse that there was something wrong. I couldn't take a full breath. The nurse chalked it up to me being nervous and gave me some Ativan. Ativan is a brand name for a tranquilizer used to treat anxiety, tension, and insomnia. It basically knocks you out! Even if you had pain, you wouldn't care. When I complained again, the nurse gave me more Ativan. (I learned to complain!) After the second shot, I didn't care that I couldn't breathe; she sent me home. All night I coughed, and coughed, and coughed to the point where my ribs began to ache. One time, I coughed so hard that I swear I passed out for a moment. I was scared. I propped all my pillows upright and began listening to my comedy tapes; I was afraid to fall asleep, I thought if I fell asleep, I could die. The first tape I listened to was Brian Regan, and I thought, If I'm going to die, I want to die laughing.

Hi, my name is Sandi Selvi. This book is about all the shit that has happened to me on my journey. It's about my life and how I've learned to laugh at everything. Now that I've been given a second chance at life, I don't want to blow it. I would like to teach you what I have learned. Without the whole lung puncture thing. There may be places where I ramble and I ramble and I ramble, and sometimes I may even repeat myself. There are also times that I may repeat myself, and places where I was too scared or sad to find the laughter. Deal with it, OK?

Comedy and family are indeed the best medicine. I've learned that laughing at my misfortune is the greatest way to deal with it. It's kind of like therapy…only cheaper. And it also gives me license to laugh at *your* misfortune. Like I tell my kids, "Don't do anything I might read about in the newspaper tomorrow." Since that didn't work, my threat is now more like, "Don't do anything you don't want to see me do on stage next week," and this goes for my friends too. They know. My comedy is about life and the things I have been through in my life.

Besides being a comedian, I have ADD (attention deficit disorder), I'm totally dyslexic, and I have multiple sclerosis (M.S.). I didn't even know what M.S. was when I was first diagnosed. So I went home from the doctor's office and Googled it. I typed in M.S.—well, actually, I typed in S&M because I'm dyslexic, and thought, "What a great disease! Now I get to wear all my black leather. This is going to be fun!" I then went out and bought a few accoutrements for my new disease. I showed up at my newly diag-nosed M.S. support group in just my thigh-highs and my ball gag, along with a few other misguided first-timers. That was when I found out, M.S./S&M…not the same thing.

So I had to find out more. I went back to the doctor and asked, "Why do I have this disease?"

"Good question…and who are you?" he asked as he scrib-bled in his notebook, not answering my question.

"How did I get this disease?" I asked with a little more authority to my voice.

"Another good question," he said, smiling, as he again wrote more furiously in his notebook.

"When did I get this disease? "

"Why did I get this disease?"

"What *is* this disease?" I demanded, grabbing the notebook out of his hand.

He looked up at me and sighed. "To answer all your ques-tions, we just don't know."

And they call themselves *specialists*. Specialists in what? Obscurity? The doctors had no real answers for me. The only thing my doctor could tell me for certain: M stands for "multiple" and S stands for "sclerosis." Thanks, Scrabble champ. I can't believe after all the years studying this stupid disease, the medical community still has no idea why some people get it, when we get it, or how we get it. I would hate to be known as a specialist in a disease about which they know absolutely nothing.

"So what are you a specialist in?"

"Nothing, and it took me an additional eight long, hard years to get here."

I'm sure their mothers are proud they paid all that money to send them through medical school to become specialists in NOTHING.

If you have M.S., you know that the disease is the result of the immune system attacking itself. The immune system is eating away at the myelin sheaths around the nerves in the brain, causing scars, sometimes lots of them. That's why they call it multiple sclerosis. "Multiple" meaning many, and "sclerosis" meaning scars. I read all this in one of the many pamphlets from the National Multiple Sclerosis Society. These scars then cause function problems, such as lack of balance, loss of sight, muscle degeneration, bladder weakness, and great cocktail party banter, you name it, depending on where they're found in the brain. I have a lot of lesions. I lost track at ten, but I know I started out with only six. I still have them. They just haven't gotten any worse since the transplant.

My first diagnosis was with the remitting/relapsing form of M.S. My symptoms were mild. Every once in a while, I would suffer a relapse, and then I would go through a period of remission. My specialist referred to these times as exacerbations. My relapses would come in the form of weakness in my left side, trembling, loss of balance and always, bladder problems. It was always either a bladder infection or I would lose bladder control. I never fully recovered, but I would come close. I could feel myself declining at a very slow rate. You know, like Mariah Carey's career. Then it would come back, like Mariah Carey's career, then go again. At first, I thought, maybe I was one of the lucky ones.

Maybe I would make it a long time without having to be in a wheelchair.

My neurologist (the *specialist*) told me about the three drugs available at the time to help slow down the progression of the disease. We called them the ABC's. Avonex, Bataseron, and Copaxon. My doctor and I decided Avonex was best for me. Except I was supposed to give myself an intramuscular shot once a week. I couldn't actually do it. Sure, I gave myself the first shot, proving to the doctor and nurse how brave I was. But did I mention it was a huge intramuscular needle? And it hurt! It hurt so bad that I couldn't do it after that first time. Everyone said it was a mental thing. No, I said, it was totally physical. It was a big fucking shot, and it hurt! So my loving husband gave me my shots from that day forward. I think he got some perverse pleasure out of it. So it was a win-win.

As if I needed more icing on the cake, nearly three years after that, I was in a car accident. The perpetrator ran a red light just as I drove into the intersection. I don't know if I was more upset about being hurt or that my car was only eleven days old. This was a setback I didn't need. The Avonex had worked pretty well up to that point, but the accident took its toll. It sent me into the worst exacerbation I had ever had—one from which I still have never fully recovered. It was like one long exacerbation that had already lasted more than two years. I began to get worse and worse. I kept experiencing every symptom I knew and a few I didn't. They showed up and stayed. I was no longer remitting.

My gait was sporadic. I never knew when my left leg was going to give me back control of my foot. I tripped a lot, it often made me appear drunk. (That's my story and I'm sticking to it.) I also had muscle spasms in my legs, arms, and back. My double vision had gone from eighteen feet to four feet. Which meant, I went from seeing anything beyond four feet as double. Oh, did I mention I had double vision? I needed a cane to walk. Sometimes I needed the cane just to find which floor was real, and other times, to just help me keep my balance. My speech was slurred, and the shaking in my hands became so erratic that I couldn't hold a pen or paintbrush. I had to give up my mural painting company, Off the Wall Designs. Life as I knew it was over. There were times I would just curl up in bed and cry. I hated being me, mostly because I was scared and had no idea what was next. I felt useless.

But even though the disease was slowly attacking my body, I wasn't going to let it kill my spirit. I got myself involved with the Silicon Valley chapter of the National Multiple Sclerosis Society in 1998. It was my way to stay on top of all the latest information. It seemed to me that the M.S. Society was getting the information faster than the doctors. Key word here: SEEMED. A year earlier, I had been voted the Mother of the Year by this chapter of the NMSS, so I knew the members were crazy. They were my kind of people. Before being nominated for Mother of the Year, I had only seen brochures about the NMSS in my doctor's office. They *seemed* (there's that word again) to have lots of information about M.S. I figured if I hung around long enough, the M.S. Society might get new information about treatments that worked. Maybe, just maybe, they could then give those *specialists* a call. They were getting new information all the time, and I wanted to be there when the cure came in.

But I was wrong. The M.S. Society only shared the same information that my doctor had. When they did get information on something the doctors thought worked, they refused to share the information and kept it to themselves for fear of lawsuits. Sure, they offered hundreds of pamphlets, telling us what we already knew: all about the symptoms, what drugs were available to slow down the progression (these pamphlets were printed by the drug companies), what diets could help some people, and what the M.S. Society offered for free to those afflicted with the disease and to their families. A trampoline was not one of them. They do help a lot of people with their programs. But the M.S.

Society was reluctant to listen about any new treatments. I know. I benefited from a new treatment, and they weren't listening to me. They feared being wrong or being sued. If the treatment was not available or affordable to "everyone," it wasn't backed by the M.S. Society. They wouldn't back anything the drug companies were against because the drug companies were backing the M.S. Society. Where was Michael Moore when I needed him?

I was taking the medications that the M.S. Society recommended, and I smoked a little pot. Someone at an M.S. support group turned me on to the fact that THC helps. The drugs the *specialists* gave me weren't working. But the pot helped a lot. I had become progressive. My M.S. wasn't slowing down at all. Unlike remitting/relapsing, when you're progressive, there's no getting back to "normal." The things that used to come back to a point stayed right where they were. Smoking pot took the edge off. The hope of me getting close to normal again was gone. I was never getting better—only worse—and things were going downhill quickly. My doctor told me that I would be in a wheelchair within five years. I kept saying to myself, "I teach tae kwan do, this can't happen to me! I'm a soccer coach. I can't be in a wheelchair." How would I wheel *that* onto a field? Then again, it could be a bonus! Anything for the team. They wouldn't throw a coach out of a game in a wheelchair. Would they? Anyway, at home I would just sit and cry. I kept thinking there were two things I did not look good in: one was green, the other was wheelchairs.

I was angry, frustrated, and scared. This beastly disease had slowly crept into my life, stealing my dreams and threatening, destroying, decaying, and corrupting everything in its path that was good, healthy, and balanced—just like my first boyfriend.

I had no idea what was going to happen to me next. I had been to see experts, specialists, and psychiatrists who dealt with M.S., and they couldn't tell me anything. Clinically, M.S. is a difficult condition to characterize because it's very unpredictable. Depending on which areas of the central nervous system are affected, and how badly they're damaged, the type and severity of symptoms can vary greatly. This means no two people get M.S. in exactly the same way. I was basically on my own.

I was a wreck, and my poor husband was trying really hard to help me deal with everything. He was something else. My M.S. was progressing so rapidly that I would have tried anything. So I did. I had almost given up hope for a normal life, when my husband met a man by chance at a meeting in January 2000. The man had to step out of the meeting to take a call from his wife. She was in the hospital. My husband asked what was wrong with her. The man said in a very matter-of-fact way, "My wife, Deb, had M.S. She went through a stem cell transplant in San Diego and is doing well, but I like to talk to her on a daily basis to see how she's getting on." My husband couldn't believe what he was hearing. *Had* M.S.? He got all the information and brought it home to me.

I looked up stem cell research on the web. Immediately, I found two articles about stem cell transplants that had been done to treat M.S. in the United States. One was about a man in Washington State who had gone through a stem cell transplant about the same time as Deb. The other was about a woman in Oregon who was already in a wheelchair, and the only thing she said was that she wished she had done it earlier. She was now getting around on her own, but felt that if she had done it earlier in her diagnosis, she would have stopped the disease and not lost so many of her functions.

I called and talked to Deb. After talking to her for an hour, my husband and I called her doctor, Dr. James Mason, at the Scripps Center in San Diego. I got back on the Internet and found that there were doctors in Italy who had been doing this to treat M.S. for more than thirty years. They all said the same thing: "M.S. is a disease where your own immune system is killing you, eating away at the myelin. This causes scarring, which interrupts your brain's normal function and causes many malfunctions of the nervous system. If you kill your immune system and build a new one, it will stop the M.S. where it is and could possibly allow your body to rebuild."

My stem cell transplant was not easy. After passing a number of tests to see if I even qualified to do the transplant, I had to then prepare myself mentally because going through this procedure meant I had to live in San Diego for two months, away from my sons. This would be very hard for me. They were young, and we had never really been apart. I love my boys. It was a tough decision. But I wanted to be around for them when they were older, so...

I was the second person in California to go through this experimental procedure called a stem cell transplant, I sometimes refer to it as a "wallet removal." Almost a hundred thousand bucks on the table. No guarantees. This was long before stem cell transplants were considered "trendy." I had it done to see if we could stop the progression of my disease. The doctors in charge of the experiment put it to me this way: "If we kill your immune system and then build you a new one, it should *theoretically* stop your M.S. from getting any worse." It didn't make any sense to me, but at the same time, somehow, it made total sense. I think this is how they built the Bionic Woman.

The scary thing is...it worked. Then President George W. Bush banned federal funding for all stem cell research. Even though there were many kinds of stem cell transplants, nobody wanted to talk about stem cells (no matter what kind). I used my own adult stem cells in a procedure called an "autologous" transplant. *Autologous*—I think it was named after a freeway in Germany. There is a happy ending to my story, because it did work. Still, nobody in a position of authority or power wanted to hear about it.

All we hear about is Bernie Madoff this, AIG that. The stock market is down; unemployment is up. Nothing in the news is good anymore. So much bad shit is happening that there is no time for fluff. Remember fluff? It was all those stupid stories that dotted the bad news with uplifting, feel-good stuff that nobody except me seems to care about anymore. I want to hear some good news for a change. I want my fluff back!

Shit happens. So much bad stuff is happening that I quit watching the news. Whatever you do, if you decide not to watch the news anymore, don't tell anyone. Before you can cover your ears, they will quickly recite all the bad shit you have been avoiding for the past month. "So then you haven't heard..." Those are now my five least-favorite words in the dictionary. They used to be "It is still your turn." That's when I played golf.

"So then you haven't heard" is usually followed by "...is dead," "...was killed," or "...in Iraq." I have had enough! Just shut up. Remember what your mother used to say: "If you don't have something nice to say, don't say anything at all." It applies here. Even Oprah has gone to the dark side. She used to have feel-good stories all the time. I could count on coming home, turning on *Oprah*, and having a good cry while I was making dinner. Now all her shows are about the money we'll be paying in taxes if my husband ever does get his bonus, how much weight I need to lose, and how unruly my kids are. My BMI is TMI. For those not in the loop, BMI is your body mass index, TMI is too much information. If I know my BMI then I can't eat what I want. Drinking is bad, nobody will let me smoke pot, and according to the doctors, no matter what we do, we're killing ourselves. Yeah, we know! Who wants to live longer anyway? Oh, that's right. Me! That's why I went through this whole stem cell thing in the first place. But I only want to live longer if you give me my fluff back! I want to hear how the guy with cancer battled back and is now doing well, how the little girl from Podunk, New York, won the spelling bee, or who it was that won the Mega Millions. I want to hear all that. Good stuff! I want to hear a feel-good story.

Here's a feel-good story for you: A woman on her fortieth

birthday began the two-month process of a stem cell transplant to combat her M.S., hoping she could do what no doctors had done for her so far and stop the progression of her disease, only to find out that it worked so well that she began to get better and better, and is now doing stand-up comedy trying to make others feel as good as she does. Nobody wants to hear that crap.

But I have written it anyway.

Chapter 1
The Tears Behind the Laughter

*I hate exercising. But my doctor says exercise, exercise, exercise.
All I heard was accessorize, accessorize, accessorize. She wants me to
get my heart rate going, so I decide to do the "Sandi Selvi" exercise
program. I smoke a cigar and drink three shots of espresso, but my
doctor didn't consider that cardio.*

Prior to my M.S. diagnosis I was practicing for my junior
black belt promotion test in tae kwon do class, when I fell. Too
dizzy to get up, I crawled to the side of the room and sat there for
a few minutes trying to regain my strength. Finally, I was able to
get up and try again. It was a spin kick with a hook, but I never
made it to the hook. I fell flat on my face. I got up feeling confused
and dizzy, yet still determined. I tried the spin kick again, only
this time, I found it harder to get back up. Lying on the floor and
feeling heavy, I tried to stand up, but couldn't. My friends gave
me some water, asked me if I was all right, and suggested that I
had been working a little too hard, striving for that black belt. The
test was that week. When I was able to stand up, I got into my car
and began to drive home.

I then realized that the left side of my face felt numb from
the top of my eyebrow to the bottom of my jawbone. It was the
strangest feeling—like Novocain gone wild. I couldn't smile
because only half of my face would respond, and my speech was
impaired. Imagine the Novocain never wearing off from the
dentist; that was how it felt. I had no idea why this was happening
or how I was ever going to eat soup again.

I went straight to the doctor. He told me the numbness might be caused by Bell's palsy, and I thought, "What does some old stripper have to do with this?" Then I found out that Bell's palsy is a disease caused by damage to the seventh cranial (facial) nerve, resulting in weakness or paralysis on one side of the face. He also said I could have a brain tumor or possibly even M.S. I knew nothing about M.S. Nor did I know anyone with M.S. I was unable to grasp just how scary it was going to get.

I never did take my tae kwon do promotion test. I never would earn my junior black belt. It was a sad ending to more than four years of hard work. I had lost my balance.

I was scared out of my mind. I had no idea what was in store for me. It just didn't sound good. I did, however, make it through a battery of other tests—the medical kind. Pee in a cup, swab this, poke that. The doctor was diligently trying to find an explanation for all the weird things that were happening to me. He used a hammer to check my reflexes, looking for weakness or overstimulation of the nerves. Sometimes the nerve endings are diminished in some places and overactive in others. After I'd undergone a brain MRI, which clearly showed six lesions, my doctor did a spinal tap to check the rate of immunoglobin (IgG). Found in the blood and lymph system, IgG antibodies fight foreign objects such as viruses, fungi, and bacteria. Most people with M.S. have elevated IgG levels. I did. I had M.S. Fuck! Fuck, fuck, fuck, fuck, fuck!

For the first few days after being diagnosed with M.S., I felt relieved. I finally could put a name to this numb face I'd been looking at for the past few weeks. It was a strange relief; the relief of knowing that something was really wrong with me. I wasn't a hypochondriac.

I wanted to know everything about this disease, multiple sclerosis. I wanted to know what it was and how to deal with it. I wanted to know it all. I wanted something to tell my friends, my family, and, especially, my children.

The doctor who diagnosed my M.S. was one of the leading neurologists in Palo Alto, a *specialist* in M.S. I was happy to know I had him to lean on and could go back to see him anytime I had questions. I began reading one of the one hundred and fifteen books I bought at the bookstore. I was trying to gather information so that I would know exactly what questions to ask my *specialist* when I saw him again, only to find out that no one really knew anything about this disease. Every book stated that it is a hard disease to define, and it's even harder to diagnose. The authors went further, explaining that everyone is affected differently. M.S. is "indefinable" and "irrational," and some books went as far as to call it a "mystery." Everything I read just upset me more.

One of the pamphlets from the doctor's office told me that "*Multiple Sclerosis* is a chronic autoimmune disease of the central nervous system in which gradual destruction of myelin occurs in patches throughout the brain or spinal cord or both, interfering with the nerve pathways and causing muscular weakness, loss of coordination, and speech and visual disturbances." It was like being drunk at a party without having any of the fun. The only real information I found about M.S. was that it affects women fifty percent more often than men. Most people with M.S. are diagnosed between the ages of twenty and forty. Stress usually plays a role in diagnosing M.S. It is rarely found in people younger than twelve or older than fifty-five, though it's not unheard of. Another fact about M.S. is that it's more common among Caucasians, especially those of Northern European ancestry. It is found more in people who live further north of the equator. Some studies show that M.S. is five times more common in North America and Europe than in the tropics.

In the United States, there is a dividing line that runs along the 37th parallel. It goes from Newport News, Virginia, all the way to Santa Cruz, California. Below the 37th parallel, the average number of cases per 100,000 people found to have M.S. is 67.5.

Above the 37th parallel, the rate is double that with 135 cases per 100,000 people. I guess I don't have to tell anyone where to buy land. What shocked me the most was that every week some two hundred people around the world are diagnosed with the disease. That's more than one person an hour. Around the world, more than 2.5 million people have the disease. Still there's no idea how or why we get it.

Angry and frustrated, I isolated myself by moving into the back bedroom of our house and began reading ferociously. I still had no idea what to tell my sons, who were only six and eight, because I had no idea what was ahead of me. I had a name to this new face of evil but no answers. I knew I was sick, but was I going to die? I read and read, getting no answers. The only thing I was getting: UPSET. My husband came running into the room to see if I was all right. He had heard the books hitting the wall.

Every book had different answers to my questions. If I didn't like what I read, I threw the book. I became so confused that I had no idea what I was going to ask the doctor. When we finally met, all I could do was ask the obvious questions: "What is this disease?" "How did I get it?" "When did I get it? " "Am I going to die from it?" Most importantly, "Are my kids going to get it?"

His answers were not the ones I wanted to hear. The only things he could tell me about the disease were the same things I had read over and over again in the books now found in a pile against the back bedroom wall. He did not say much, but I swear I heard him mumble "Shit happens" as he left the examination room.

M.S. is an autoimmune disease, which means that my immune system was attacking itself. Sure, I could read about the symptoms, but why? I was living them. In less than six months my symptoms had spread from the numbness in half my face, to needing a cane to walk, to suffering muscle spasms from my neck down my back and into my legs. The *specialist* couldn't answer my questions. With all the studies and all the specialists in the world, they have failed to explain anything about this disease. They don't know. They especially didn't have the answer to my most important question: Is it hereditary? Are my boys going to get it too? They couldn't tell me what symptoms were in my future and when I would die from it. Oh! But they did know one thing: More than likely I was going to die from it. One of the symptoms would get me in the end.

Maybe it would be dehydration and malnutrition from the inability to swallow, or kidney failure (because kidney problems are common in M.S. due to the high rate of urinary tract infections). That I knew. Or it could be by choking or aspiration, because the throat muscles could stop working, causing me to choke on food. Read that too! I could aspirate food or a drink, causing pneumonia. Or my favorite: the consequences of inactivity, which includes infected bedsores, stasis pneumonia, or a heart attack. And last but not least: suicide. M.S. can cause depression, and depression can lead to suicide. Roughly three percent of people with M.S. commit suicide. After finding out all this information, I could see why people with M.S. are depressed! With all the obscurities, just knowing they have M.S. could send anyone over the edge.

I went into the biggest bout of depression I had ever experienced. I sat around for weeks, trying to decipher the books, the disease, and life. I began having trouble talking. Sometimes I would go to say something to someone, and it would sound like I had been drinking, or I had the word in my mouth, but couldn't say it right no matter how hard I tried. Then I couldn't remember words. Months later, I started losing control of my bladder. I barely made it home one afternoon. I ran to the bathroom and didn't get my pants down in time. That was a good day. At least I was not at the corner of Cox and Saratoga Avenue. Again. The tremors in my hands worsened every day. I could no longer paint, which took the fun out of having my own painting business. That was also my creative outlet at the time. With all my new symptoms, I physically couldn't do anything I really wanted to do. More importantly, as my symptoms worsened, I couldn't do the things I needed to do.

My husband and I agreed that we had to be as honest with our children as we could. It was obvious that I was ill. They weren't stupid. We told them what we knew. Of course, they too wanted to know if I was going to die. My sons would go to our friends' or family members' homes to give me a break, and within a few hours, they wanted to come home and check on me. I would just lie in my bed and cry. I felt useless. I didn't feel like I was doing such a great job being a mom.

My mom, on the other hand, was awesome. She would come over and help me with the chores, and she would sometimes take the boys for a few hours to give me a break. I remember crying and telling her how much M.S. sucked. She always told me that no matter how bad it seemed, there was always someone out there who had it worse off than you. Then she said, "You could have a child with this disease." She paused and smiled. "See, I have it worse off than you." She was sad, but she always seemed to say just the right thing to make me feel better. She and I spent a lot of time together. My father had remarried and was living in Palm Springs. When he called from time to time, I could hear in his voice that he was as sad as my mother. M.S. affected everyone around me.

The worse my symptoms got, the less I could do. We had purchased season passes to the Boardwalk in Santa Cruz and Great America theme park for my boys, my nephew, and me every year since they were toddlers. After a while, our weekly trips to Great America and Santa Cruz during the summer became just one trip all season. That was hard on all of us. I could no longer do the things I wanted. Things had definitely changed.

I was getting more symptoms. I lost my balance. Walking became difficult, but the heat affected me the most. In extreme

heat, I could barely walk. I could only go a few steps without tripping or falling. My feet felt like lead. I began using a cane all the
time. The kids were embarrassed when I pulled it out. Then I realized it was always missing. When I asked about it, my husband
told me he was storing it in the garage for me. Even he was embarrassed. No one wanted to look at it. It was a constant reminder.

The worse I became, the harder it got on my family. I know
it was difficult for them, watching me go from an energetic mom
who did everything from teaching art at their school, to coaching
their soccer and basketball teams, to playing games with them
every chance I could—all before making a home-cooked meal
every evening—to this person who could no longer speak without
slurring her words or hold a brush to paint. The worst thing was
every time we got on a plane to go on a vacation, or even on a
short trip, I would get sick as a dog.

When I drove, I couldn't tell the distance between my car
and the car in front of me. The double vision was getting worse.
I was in several small fender benders. Driving became a luxury
for emergencies only. I became dependent on my friends. But I
could tell it was weighing heavily on them too. They found it hard
to see me like that. I used to do everything for myself, but with this
disease, some days I wouldn't have been able to get out of bed
even if the house were on fire. I knew it was hard for them to call
and hear all about my constant problems. I knew because the
phone stopped ringing.

My family and friends rarely stopped by, and when they did,
the looks on their faces made me feel worse than if they hadn't
stopped by at all. I began getting all too familiar with what I called
the "pity" look. The "pity" look was a combination of someone
on the verge of tears, and ready to mutter the words "Bless your
heart." My grandmother would say "Bless your heart" when she
saw a really ugly baby or when she knew someone was dying.

I didn't want pity. I just wanted people to understand that
I was the same person inside; I just couldn't do the things they

were used to seeing me do. Things had changed so much that I was beyond pity. Shit had not already happened. It had hit the fan. I was quickly approaching the "Bless your heart" stage, and even I knew it. I had quit working, quit playing golf, quit coaching, and quit practicing tae kwon do. I had just quit. I, like so many of my friends and family, saw my life quickly sinking into a black hole, except I didn't have the luxury of not coming by and pretending the M.S. wasn't there. I was living with it.

Shit happens!

All I could think was that luckily for my family—but unluckily for me—most people who have M.S. do not live past their sixties. Unluckily for my family and me, people who have this disease cannot live independently or comfortably. Shit! Reality sucks. The more I read, the more frightened I became. Someone is eventually going to have to take care of me. Just put me in a home now! I don't expect anyone to take care of me. No one signed up for this shit, especially not me.

My support group had dwindled to a small number of close friends. I was spending more time in bed and less time with the boys. They were getting more anxious as the time passed. We all were. My husband seemed to be holding strong, but, I could tell he was getting tired of hearing all of the bad stuff every day. He was there, not as much as I would have liked, but he was there. I couldn't even imagine what he was going through with a sick wife and two small children at home. His work was demanding more of his time. Coincidentally, the more time he spent at work, the worse I got. When he was there, he was the glue.

Every time I had a small problem, I would head back to the doctor. The visits were becoming more and more frequent. The list of symptoms continued to grow. I no longer had control of my bladder. It wasn't just the heat that affected me anymore; now the extreme cold took its toll. One night, I was walking down the hall, and when my feet hit the cold marble floor, the muscles in my legs cramped up so tight that I fell down. The cold from the marble penetrated me to the bone. I couldn't move. Every muscle in my body froze, and all I could do was lie there in a heap on the floor. I couldn't say a word, all I could do was whimper. It took my husband a few minutes to realize I wasn't in bed. When he came down the hall looking for me, there I was lying on the floor. He got tears in his eyes. He quickly scooped me up and carried me into the bedroom, put me under the covers, and turned the electric blanket on high. He rubbed me all over to warm me up. When I saw the panicked look in his eyes, I grew more frightened.

I was so scared and had no idea what was in store next. Kind of like being in a terrifying limbo, I was in fear for myself and my family. My life had completely changed. I no longer recognized it.

I would have done anything to stop, slow down, or obliterate M.S.—I even went as far as wearing a "Cold Suit." My friend's neighbor knew a guy, who knew a guy (this sounds like the beginning of a bad joke, or a mob hit) who introduced me to a man at NASA, Bill Elkins. This was the guy who invented THE space suit, the one the astronauts wore. This guy was smart, a true rocket scientist. My new friend Bill had just invented a suit for you to wear that kept your core temperature more even. It helped stop my muscle spasms, it took my double vision away, and it just felt good. The only problem—it was a tad cumbersome and ugly.

The cold suit consisted of a bright cobalt blue jacket with matching cap that reminded me of one a jockey would wear. And, I swear it glowed in the dark. But, not only was it ugly, it was attached by hoses to a small cooler that had to be filled with ice. At first I thought it was a joke. If he had been around back then, I would have been searching again for Ashton Kutcher. But the damn thing worked. To this day I don't know what happened to Bill and his company.

Chapter 2
My Theories about M.S.

It's the same thing Annette Funicello has. You know her; she was in the Mickey Mouse Club and in the Beach Blanket Bingo *movie. She was the one who did that dance. It turns out that wasn't a dance. Those were tremors.*

I have my own theories about M.S. There is mass confusion in the medical industry, among doctors in particular. Nobody has answers. I know firsthand. Looking back throughout the years, so many weird things have happened to me that I'm wondering if I have the answers to why I have it. Maybe there's a connection between some unfortunate incidents and my affliction with this disease.

I grew up in and around San Jose, California. We lived in Campbell—in the 37th parallel—until I was about five years old. Our house sat on a quaint, tree-lined court. The kids in our neighborhood were all about the same ages as my older brother and me. We all hung out in the court together (this was back when playing in the front yard was still considered safe). Everybody knew each other, and we watched out for each other, except for one kid whom we tied to a tree, but he had it coming.

As a child, I was allergic to nearly everything in my front yard, except the mailbox. I couldn't go outside without having to use an inhaler, or I'd end up being rushed to the doctor for a shot. When it was our turn to have all the neighborhood kids over to our house, I couldn't go out front to play with them as they climbed on the branches of our walnut tree or wrestled on the lawn. I was allergic. All I could do was watch them anxiously from my bedroom window. I would rest my chin or bite down on the windowsill as I watched them play in my yard, every once in a while taking a break to suck on my inhaler.

My asthma and allergies were so bad that a nurse came to our house and gave me a shot every morning on her way to work. I felt like John Belushi. My nurse, Mrs. Aroldie, lived two doors down from us. Every day on her way to work she would stop by our house where I would be hiding in the opening at the bottom of the linen closet with my butt hanging out. And *every day* she would say in a loud, questioning voice, "Where is Sandi? I guess if we can't find her she won't have to have her shot today." She would come to the closet, open the door, pull my pants down, give me my shot, and then close the closet door. I could hear her talking to my mother about all kinds of things before they said their goodbyes, and then she was off to work. Then when my mother would tell me it was safe to come out, I would climb out of the closet and shyly laugh. "Got her again."

My mother would always tell me that I had missed out on Mrs. Aroldie and how they were surprised they couldn't find me. I would skip down the hall back to my room and go on with my day like nothing happened. *Denial*, it's not just a lake in Pittsburgh or something like that. But there were those few days I happened to be around when she came over. It wasn't the same. I didn't make it into the linen closet, and the charade was off. Those shots hurt like hell. I would cry and rub the sore spot all day, feeling sorry for myself. Those days I hated Mrs. Aroldie. The other days I just loathed her.

THEORY #1 *for why I think I have M.S.*

Could it be from all the shots I had as a child? Were they really good for me? Maybe Mrs. Aroldie was a witch and cast a spell, and when I say "witch," I am being kind.

While standing by my window and watching with envy as my friends rode their bikes down the street, I would bite down on the windowsill and rest my head. Oh my God, I ate lead paint as a child!

THEORY #2 *for why I think I have M.S.*

Could it have been from the lead paint on the windowsill? In 1964, lead paint was common. I chewed and gnawed on the windowsill out of pure frustration. I was stuck on the inside looking out at my friends playing without me. It was the perfect picture of youth, and I couldn't be a part of it. I was pathetic. I ate windowsills for breakfast, lunch, and dinner. I chewed a beautifully scalloped design into those silly sills. It was artistic. Or at least that's the way I saw it. My parents only saw the damage. They couldn't see my artistic ability—how each bite was placed so carefully and deliberately.

My father was furious. In order to get me out of the house, he decided to build me a playhouse in the backyard, away from the walnut tree, grass, and *especially* windowsills. The playhouse was every girl's dream. It had windowsills everywhere! I could chew and gnaw till my heart was content, and no one would yell at me. It was my house. There was only one thing missing in my perfect home—the husband to do all the cooking.

As soon as the playhouse was fully constructed, my father sent me out to inspect his handiwork. I walked all around, peeking in each window and opening and closing each door. Wow, my very own house! It was the coolest thing I had ever seen.

"OUCH! What was that?" Seriously, that hurt! One of the first things I did while investigating my new home was step on a nail, and I thought allergy shots hurt! Nails hurt a lot more than any shot. Needles don't seem so big now.

My mother called the doctor to tell him that I had stepped on a nail, and he told her to find the nail to make sure it wasn't rusty, or if it was, I would need a tetanus shot. The whole family went out back to look for the nail. I led the search and told them it was on a flat board sticking straight up, not easy to see. It was somewhere behind the house. I was sure of it. I looked for what seemed like hours and became so tired that I could no longer stand. So I found a flat board to sit on, hoping to get a better perspective on things.

"OUCH! What was that?" I sat right on it this time! Everyone laughed at me. We rushed to the doctor's office with nail in hand, or butt. And yes, it was rusty.

NOTE TO SELF: Tetanus shots hurt more than rusty nails, and rusty nails hurt more than allergy shots. No need to hide from Mrs. Aroldie anymore.

THEORY #3 *for why I think I have M.S.*

Rusty nails and a tetanus shot at such an early age could not have been good for me. Could they be the cause of my M.S.?

Sure, lockjaw would've been worse than the shot, but not according to some. My brother, always telling me to shut up, would have loved it if I had lockjaw. Speaking of my brother…he's the reason for theories #4–6, starting with him putting a straw into the gas tank of our neighbor's car. Ever since the gasoline incident at the age of two, my hatred for cars has just grown. I have always hated cars. This is what happened: one day my brother put a straw into the tank of the car and convinced me that it would be a good idea to take a sip. He was my big brother, and I idolized him. I would have done anything he said. Okay! I *did* everything he said. He swore it would taste good, and I believed him. So I wanted more than a sip. I wanted a Big Gulp o' Gas. Big Gulp o' Gas equals stomach pumping at the hospital.

So I seriously hate cars. I hate driving them, I hate wrecking them, and the smell of gasoline still makes me gag.

The only things I've learned about cars since the age of two:

1. "E" means empty, not almost empty. If it meant almost empty, there would be an "A" there.

2. After five months, foil-wrapped chicken, even if it's still wrapped in foil, will make your car smell unbearable.

3. If you are making out with a guy and kick a car out of gear, it will roll down the hill and take out your neighbor's mailbox, his fence, and then the neighbor if he doesn't get out of the way—and you had better put your bra back on.

4. If you see a car take out your mailbox and then your fence, get the fuck out of the way.

5. No matter what your brother says, gasoline does not taste good.

THEORY #4 *for why I think I have M.S.*

Doctors made me swallow charcoal to absorb the gasoline because they didn't want me to throw up the gasoline and cause more damage to my throat. Then they pumped my stomach to get it all out. Neither the charcoal nor the gasoline, with all its chemicals, could have been good for me. Could this be why I have M.S.?

Soon after that, we went to visit my dad's friend from the police department. He and his wife had two kids who were younger than my brother and me. We grew bored quickly of the See n' Say and tried to find things to do. My brother dragged me into their garage and tricked me into swallowing some ant poison that was hidden under the workbench behind a box of nails. I thought, "Gee, he was so right about the gasoline." Shit happens.

THEORY #5 *for why I think I have M.S.*

Who knows what was in that poison? If it can kill an ant, it wasn't good.

Another visit to the emergency room to get my stomach pumped. Another day of horrid visions of doctors sticking their fingers down my throat was etched in my mind forever thanks to my brother.

THEORY #6 *for why I think I have M.S.*

Maybe my brother frazzled my nerves so much when I was a child that he caused me permanent nerve damage.

Chapter 3
What Is M.S.?

When I was first diagnosed with multiple sclerosis, the doctor actually gave me medical marijuana, and my insurance paid for it. That's when I realized there is a God.

After many years, I checked myself into rehab, and that same insurance company, the one that paid for my marijuana, wouldn't pay for my rehab.

So, then I began to wonder: was my M.S. due to something that happened to me after we had moved? When I was five years old, we moved to the New Almaden area of San Jose—still in the 37th parallel. Our house was on a six-block-square housing development called Montevideo at the end of Camden Avenue. That was when Camden Avenue was a dead-end street, back in the '60s. Redmond, Camden, and Coleman bordered my new neighborhood. The new neighborhood was very similar to my old neighborhood in Campbell because everyone knew each other except in this neighborhood we had apricot and cherry trees, but thank God no walnut trees. It was larger, however. But I was larger too (or so I thought). I *was* five!

This home was on a long narrow L-shaped street. And there were kids, at least thirty of them. On our half of the street alone, there were kids of all ages. And more kids lived on the other streets surrounding our street. It seemed like there were thousands of them.

I quickly made friends. It wasn't hard. There were kids everywhere, and if you didn't fit in one place, you could always go next door. Or to the next door, or the next. There was always someone somewhere, wanting to do something.

Some families that had only one kid seemed strange to me. It was the first time I had ever met a family with only one child before. Then I met several families with teenagers *and* babies. I figured they had the older kids to baby-sit the younger ones. Smart! Then there were the families I had to investigate more closely. Those were the ones with five or more kids. How did they do it? I had never seen that before either. Boy, did that fascinate me. Our family could hardly keep it together with just two kids, and these families seemed to be doing great with five, six, or even seven kids.

One of my best friends, Judy, came from one of these *big* families. I totally envied her because she always had someone to talk to. Always! And she got to share a room with her two sisters, while I was always alone. She said she hated it because she never had a moment alone and *always* had people around her. She envied my peace and the fact that I had a room to myself. Both my parents worked; my brother was always off. I hated being alone. I couldn't believe two people could see the same thing so differently.

Judy and I spent a lot of time together. We had our first communion together and beat up the neighborhood bully together. We were a team. We had dances in her garage, and her mother taught me how to burp. Hey, it could have been worse. We started out playing with our Barbies when we were little, and at the age of thirteen, we learned to smoke together. Life was fun back then. It was easy.

THEORY #7-8 *for why I think I have M.S.*

Smoking cigarettes? Or Barbie!

It couldn't have been Barbie. She was plastic. But there was no such thing as carcinogens back then *and* she was my friend.

We played dress-up together. Nobody would put dangerous things in toys. And it couldn't have been the cigarettes because the tobacco companies told us they weren't bad. And everybody I knew smoked. None of them have M.S.

Montevideo was fun. It was a great place to be in the late '60s and early '70s. There's even a Facebook page, "I Grew Up in Montevideo in the 1970s." We would all hang out at the pool with our cigarettes. If we ran out, Nanci, my crazy next-door neighbor and first comedy mentor, would put her mom's wig on and go to the 7-Eleven and get some more. If we weren't at the pool, we were at a local apricot orchard, where we would all work cutting apricots for pennies a crate.

THEORY #9 *for why I think I have M.S.*

The apricots could have been covered in pesticides! Could it be the pesticides? We all went to a farm right outside our subdivision of Montevideo and literally stood for hours cutting apricots in half and putting the pits in a pail.

We could ride our bikes all over the development and never get lost. If we were brave enough, we would even go exploring in the foothills or down to the creek. The bridge scared me though because one day a truck came by as we were walking, and Judy's sister moved so close to the edge, she fell off the bridge and into the creek. We were all afraid to go down there after that.

THEORY #10 *for why I think I have M.S.*

The Guadalupe Creek flowed passed the Guadalupe mines. It was well known for being full of metals, especially mercury. We played there all the time as children. Could this be it? My reason for having multiple sclerosis?

Even though the Guadalupe mines were fairly close, nobody ever rode up Guadalupe Mines Road. The reason? People always told stories about a crazy man with a hook for a hand, who waited until dark, then came out and took children. I know this story because I was one of the ones who told it over and over again to all the little kids in the neighborhood.

We would try to scare each other by telling stories about that crazy man sneaking up on cars at night and scaring people to death. One story was about a couple who heard a noise and raced away, only to get home to find a bloody hook attached to their door handle. We told the stories so often that we all began to believe them. So we never went up there again.

At the other end of the development, there was a huge old brown house. The shutters were falling off, and the paint was chipping off of the eaves and gutters. There was an old tree out front that looked like a tree out of a scary story. Its branches were black with mold, and the leaves were small and white and glistened in the moonlight. It was a spooky house. And it smelled like old sneakers. We were all afraid to go near it. But one day when we were passing by, my friend pushed me into the front yard. I fell down and was covered with stinging nettles, and I smelled like mold.

THEORY #11-12 *for why I think I have M.S.*

Do stinging nettles have anything to do with multiple sclerosis? What about mold?

An old man from inside the spooky house came out and yelled, "GO! Git away from here, or the tree will grab you!" That was when I realized, if you looked at the tree from the right angle, it looked just like a hand reaching out of the ground about ready to tear the door right off the front of the house. Or grab me. Then I heard a dog bark. I was petrified. I swear I wet my pants. I could hardly move, but I got up and ran anyway. I'm convinced he was standing on the porch waving goodbye to me with a hook where his hand should have been. I was so scared, but never went that way again to see for sure.

Across the street from us lived a man who, until he was caught, was a bank robber. We had no idea. He was called the "Columbo Bank Robber," because he wore a hat and trench coat into the banks he robbed. He looked just like Columbo on TV.

He seemed like such a nice guy, and he was so handsome. I baby-sat for him and his wife all the time. They had two sons. The Bank Robber was one of my father's closest friends. They had a group of guys in the neighborhood that played poker together. But the bank robber shot and killed himself on his last heist. His death really shook my family and our neighborhood. Judy and I still talk about it to this day as if it just happened yesterday. It was such a tragedy. He left behind a wife and two small children. He also left a neighborhood of stunned parents and children of all ages wondering what happened. Back then, no one was allowed to talk about it; it was too weird to talk about. He was dead, that was enough. But an endless stream of onlookers drove past the house where the "Columbo Bank Robber" once lived. That gave us kids something to do: stare at the cars and sell Columbo T-shirts.

I can't imagine how my father felt when he found out one of his best friends was a bank robber. "Why?" you ask. Because my father was a cop. And he wasn't just any cop, he ended up being the chief of police of San Jose.

Yeah, I was a bit of a local celebrity. Sure, the other kids avoided me like the plague. But they knew me! And by the way, do you know how hard it is to get a date when your father is a cop? Oh, sorry, the chief of police? The only thing harder…getting drugs! Hey, it was the '70s.

THEORY #13 *for why I think I have M.S.*

Drugs. I wonder if those drugs had anything to do with my M.S.? Nahh!

We lived in Almaden where I remained until the middle of

my sophomore year at Branham High School. Then my father decided to remove us from crime-infested and drug-riddled San Jose. He dropped us in the middle of the San Lorenzo Valley in the Santa Cruz Mountains. Better known as Ben Lomond, California, it was a pot smokers' paradise—still in the 37th parallel.

I had just recently won the 1976 Miss Teen San Jose pageant, and I was going to Newport Beach over the summer for the state finals. All the girls at my school hated me, so moving to a new town was a blessing for me. I was moving to my new town with a clean slate. No one knew me, and I could just be me. I was *not* a cop's daughter, and I was *not* Miss Teen San Jose. No one there could hold anything against me because they didn't know me yet.

On my first day at San Lorenzo Valley High School, I thought I would go undetected. I checked in at the office, got my schedule, and went off to my first class. The second I arrived the teacher announced, "Everyone, this is Sandi. She's the new girl you've all been hearing about." All I could think was "WHAT? Hearing about?"

Then the teacher laid the local newspaper on the desk in front of me. I was horrified. There it was. The headline read, in the biggest, boldest letters they could find, "SLVHS WELCOMES MISS TEEN SAN JOSE!" Right under the headline was a picture that will haunt me forever. The picture was of me, with my mouth wide open, and a woman standing behind me pinning a tiara on top of my head as I was being handed a bouquet of flowers. I looked around the room; everyone just stared. FUCK! Not so undetected. Bad day to wear my tiara.

I spent a lot of time at San Lorenzo Valley High School hiding from the local girls, who liked to beat up skinny blonde bitches who came from "Over the Hill." They thought I was invading their space and trying to take their men. Like I would have wanted any of their socially inept mountain thugs. "Over the Hill" is usually a phrase reserved for people in their 50s, but in Santa Cruz County, "Over the Hill" refers to anyone from the

San Jose side of Highway 17. Basically the whole Bay Area. And there were a lot of girls who hated anyone from "Over the Hill." I know every one of them.

I finally found a few misfits to hang out with, who've stayed my lifelong friends. We called ourselves the IBTC (The Itty Bitty Titty Committee). We had T-shirts printed and everything. We did everything together. Our leader was Amber. Pretty menacing name, don't you think? She was the leader for all the apparent reasons. Number one: her titties were not itty bitty at all. She must have been at least a 38D. Number two: if she wasn't the leader, she would've beaten the shit out of us. So she was the president of the club. (There's nothing more embarrassing than getting beat up by an Amber.)

We would drive down to the Santa Cruz Beach Boardwalk almost every weekend. There we would cruise on the main drag. I would drive my VW Bug with Amber in the passenger seat next to me, with Kim in the back right next to Cathy. My other friends, Stacy and Patti, were in their cars next to us. Without fail, as soon as we passed a bunch of good-looking guys, Amber would knock my car out of gear. The engine would rev out of control, and they would all point and laugh at me. She would just smirk. I would laugh and swear I would get her back, but I never did.

The first time I smoked pot was with my IBTC gang, and the first time I got drunk was with them too. We basically grew up together doing the teen things that every parent fears. But drinking really wasn't my thing, so I became the designated driver for such outings. That is, until graduation; that's when it was my turn.

Amber and I had arrived at the meeting place. It was a point at the end of a street up in the mountains, where we were all going to meet after we picked up what we wanted to drink for the evening. We had all graduated from high school, and we were going to *celebrate*. We bought sloe gin. It tasted horrible, but we chugged it down anyways. Okay, I chugged it down. I plugged my nose and swallowed. I passed the bottle to Amber, and she took a sip, and then she passed it back to me. I plugged my nose, gulped down as much as I could before I had to take a breath, and then I passed it back to her, and she took a sip. I gulped. She sipped. In no time, I was wasted. I had never felt like that before. I could barely stand up on my own. I liked it. Being falling-down drunk was kind of fun. Little did I know that years later I would have given anything to be able to stand up on my own.

When it was time to drive home, I couldn't do it. I was trying to put the house key in my car's ignition. I couldn't understand why my house wouldn't start. Amber put me in the passenger seat and drove me home. She had a friend of ours follow her so that he could drive her home from there. She planted me on the porch with my key in my hand and told me to wait until they were gone before entering the house. They ran down the driveway and drove off. I spent the next twenty-five minutes trying to stop swaying long enough to put the key in the lock so that I could unlock the door and get in the house. I must have made a racket hitting the door with my key because the next thing I knew, it flew open on its own. My father was just standing there. I fell on my face. He reached down, picked me up, and in his not so fatherly cop voice asked, "Where have you been?" I began to explain, "Me and Amber—"

He interrupted and corrected me, "It's 'Amber and I.'"

I so stupidly and innocently corrected him right back. "You weren't there."

The only thing I remember hearing after that was the word "grounded," repeated over and over again. Sure, there were other words said before it and after it, but none were pronounced so clearly. And I was grounded. For a whole week. I couldn't do anything. Good thing, because that was how long my hangover lasted.

San Lorenzo Valley High was, and still is, located in a tiny town called Felton, California. The kids who went there came from all the surrounding little towns—from Boulder Creek, to Ben Lomond, and even as far up as Bonnie Doon—all towns that make up the San Lorenzo Valley in the Santa Cruz Mountains.

What I am finding out now about this area is that it's a hotbed of multiple sclerosis. You know how I explained the 37th parallel? Santa Cruz is the westernmost ending point across the U.S., just a few minutes' drive from the San Lorenzo Valley. And I believe the San Lorenzo Valley is weird. It's an area with its own little parallel.

With the United States population being roughly 306 million people, the incident rate of multiple sclerosis is about 350,000. That means that the average is approximately 11 people per 10,000 are diagnosed with M.S. San Lorenzo Valley High School had an average of 150 students per graduating class in the '70s and early '80s. I have personally found 13 people in the graduating classes from 1975 to 1980 who have M.S. With less than 1,000 people, that's more than ten times the national average. WOW! ...WHY?

Interesting, huh? Back to my story...I worked in the same shopping center as my friend Kim from the backseat of the VW. I worked for my mother. My mom was awesome. She owned the cutest dress shop in Aptos, California. It was called Dress Rehearsal. I tried to help her manage it for years. Okay, I was in it for the clothes. I took them instead of a paycheck. My friend Kim worked for the shoe store right across the hall, Shoe Biz. She basically did the same. She had more shoes than Imelda Marcos. I remember one month Kim had to borrow money, she owed her boss at the end of a pay cycle. It wasn't our fault there were no customers. There was nothing to do. We were bored. We were either shopping or calling each other to complain about how bored we were. Our boredom would quickly turn into games, and we would try to trick each other on the phone by disguising our voices.

It was something to do.

One day I called Kim pretending to be deaf. There was not a living soul in the entire shopping center, and I didn't know what to do with myself. I was just sitting at the desk staring at the phone, so I called Kim and asked, "Do you sell shoes?" But in such a voice that it came out more like "Duh ya tell choose?"

Kim was mortified. She didn't know what to say, because she couldn't understand me.

"What?" she said, so sweetly.

"Ant ya a choo stow?" I asked impatiently.

"Are we a shoe store?" she repeated. "Why, yes, we are."

"Dank joo, bye-bye," and I hung up.

Within a few minutes, my phone rang and a voice said, "Duh joo tell close?"

I said, "Hi, Kim!"

"How did you know it was me?" she said with such surprise.

"I dun nuh, I get I an smar," I answered.

"That was you?"

After that we couldn't even look at each other without tears rolling out of our eyes. We were both bored stiff (and sick in the head), but we continued to use that voice for months and find ways to amuse ourselves. Every time we called each other, we would inquire whether the other sold shoes or clothes in that voice. It kept us busy. Then my mother hired a girl to work for her and me. I had to train her. After teaching her to check new clothes in, straighten up the racks, and close the books for the day, I made her learn the voice. I was a special kind of evil.

THEORY #14 *for why I think I have M.S.*

This must be payback for being such a brat. Karma's a bitch.

I had the new girl call Kim pretending to be me asking if she sold shoes (in the voice), while I stood outside Kim's store. As soon as I heard Kim's patent answer, "No, wee dun tell choose no mow," I walked in and with a confused look on my face asked her who she was talking to. She panicked and hung up the phone. I almost wet my pants. And if this is not why I have M.S., it is definitely why I am going to hell.

After goofing off with Kim all summer, I started school at San Jose State University, trying to make a life for myself. I hated school, but I knew that I needed to finish. I had read somewhere that people were happier if they had a college degree. I wanted to be happy. I continued working with my mom, going on buying trips and staying in school full time.

I didn't know it, but I had experienced my first M.S. symptom during my freshman year of college. During my first set of finals, I was under a lot of stress. I had what is referred to as an "exacerbation." An exacerbation is a term I have become very familiar with, and have learned to hate. An exacerbation is when the symptoms of M.S. flare up. It could be a different kind of flare up every time. One or all of your M.S. symptoms get really bad; they become very pronounced, and then, when the "exacerbation" is over, they disappear.

I had a pain in my stomach that made me feel sick. It hurt so much that whenever I touched my stomach, I would throw up. The pain was sharp and low to the right. It was near my appendix, but *this* pain wrapped around to the back and felt like someone had put a girdle on me, but cinched it way too tight. My boyfriend at the time rushed me to the school doctor. The doctor took one look at me and had me rushed to the local hospital. The local hospital did blood tests and seemed baffled, but they decided that it was indeed my appendix, and it had to go.

Within a few hours, I was sedated and lying in bed, feeling great—just like every Friday night. Then my father came in. He is where I get my sense of humor. Only this wasn't so funny: the week before the "appendix incident" he had taken my friend Patti and me to see the movie *Coma*. If you haven't seen it, or read the book, this will make no sense. But my father came running into my room in a complete panic and said very quietly, "I'll go check the pipes." Then he ran out.

See, in *Coma*, the main character was going into surgery to have his appendix removed. He was so heavily sedated he couldn't tell anyone that the doctors were actually piping in gas (instead of oxygen) to be used during surgery. He figured out that this was why all the people going into surgery were coming out in comas. And then the doctors were selling their body parts! "I'll go check the pipes" was the last line the guy heard before he went completely under. My father thought his joke was funny, but when he came back into the room to tell me he was just kidding, there I was, on the floor, trying to put my pants on so I could run. Hilarious!

Then my doctors took out a perfectly good appendix, explaining, "Wow, and we totally thought when the tests came up negative, they were wrong." Again, hilarious! And these weren't even *specialists*. I, along with the hole in my body where my appendix used to be, went back to school that week and took three of five finals I had for the semester. Two of my teachers felt sorry for me and excused me from their finals. The rest hardly even noticed I was gone.

I never had quite the severity of problems that I had that one semester, but I did feel quite fatigued for the rest of my days in college. That had to have been from taking all my classes on Tuesdays and Thursdays and working full-time to help pay for school. It wasn't the partying, the men, the drugs, or the pot.

Chapter 4
It's Getting Worse

My father was the chief of police of San Jose. He used to intimidate my dates. He would ask for fingerprints, blood, and a copy of their driver's license before I was allowed to go out with them. I used to tell him to just wait until the end of the date, and I would have their entire DNA. But finally I found Mr. Right. Well, 'Mr. Always Thinks He's Right.' My dad was funny. He would kill mosquitoes and rats because he was afraid of them spreading disease, and yet he let my first boyfriend live.

I met my husband Rob during my senior year in college when I was healthy (other than the appendix thing). He lived next door to a guy I was tutoring. During my last two years at San Jose State, I was supposed to work on the school paper. But being on the paper meant being at school five days a week. I couldn't do that since I was working full-time.

I talked to the dean of journalism, and he told me that all I needed to do was tutor someone in advertising instead of working on the paper. That would fulfill my obligation. So I began tutoring this guy named Craig with his advertising homework every Thursday night. He was a really nice guy. He lived in a duplex in Campbell with his wife and daughter. He was so sweet to me. He was always trying to set me up with guys.

He worked at a shop called the Sports Fan, where he met all the local athletes at autograph signings and charity functions. He often dragged me along. He introduced me to some of the 49ers, some of the A's, and a few of the Giants. But I liked the football players.

Then, in my last semester of school, Craig introduced me to Rob, who lived right next door to him and looked like a football player. It turns out he played football in high school and college. Craig had mentioned Rob a few times and told me I would like him, but I thought Craig was kind of strange—sweet but strange. He referred to his neighbor Rob as his friend, and I really didn't want to know his friends. So I put off meeting Rob for months.

One day, I was sitting on the porch, waiting for my tutee to show up, when up drove this extremely good-looking huge guy in a shiny red Mustang convertible. He was wearing a blue baseball cap on backwards, and his smile was kind through his thick bushy mustache. He approached me in an awkward, but cute way. He told me he had just gotten off work from Apple Computer, and our first conversation began.

"What are you doing here?" he asked.

"I'm Craig's tutor, and I'm waiting for him to arrive," I replied.

"YOU'RE Craig's tutor?" he asked in surprise.

Then the two of us sat talking on the porch for what seemed like hours. Turns out he felt the same way I did about meeting anyone my tutee, Craig, considered a friend. It turned out Craig had told him all about me too, but he was just as leery. When Craig finally showed up for his lesson, he was so frazzled that he didn't want to do schoolwork. Turns out he had problems at work that afternoon, which was why he was late.

Rob, Craig, and I sat and watched Cheers, which became our show. As soon as it was over, Rob walked me to my car. We made out for half an hour and then made a date to meet the following Thursday night to watch Cheers again. I am such a slut. This went on for quite some time. He would meet me at Craig's after our tutoring session, and we would all watch Cheers. Afterward, Rob would walk me to my car, we would make out for a long time, and then I would drive home—alone. Finally, one evening he asked me out for a real date.

He came over to Santa Cruz to pick me up. I was living at home at the time. My parents had sold the mountain house and were living in a pristine white condo, exactly 1.2 miles from the beach, in Santa Cruz, California. Rob picked me up and took me out for a really elegant dinner. Then he wanted to go to the beach. He had brought champagne, but I didn't like to drink. He seemed very disappointed. Here he'd planned this romantic evening sipping champagne, under the moonlight, on the beach, and I had to say, "No, I don't drink. Thanks anyways!" I thought we had a good time! But I didn't hear from him all week.

The following week, Craig and his wife were having a Halloween party. Craig told me that Rob was going to be there. I was so nervous. I had to find something to dress up as, that would be cute, but not too slutty. It had to be smart, but not so smart that no one got it.

I dressed up as a green M&M. Everyone knew that green M&M's made you horny. I thought that was a great way to get his attention. I showed up at the party. Two hours later Rob still wasn't there. Finally at about 10:30, I began to melt, so I left. There I was, sitting in my car, when he drove up with another girl. She was dressed as a cheerleader, and we all know how they like to drink; I didn't stand a chance. They entered Rob's house. The lights went on, the lights went off. I drove home alone.

Craig told him how upset I was. He called the next day to explain that he had made that date way before we even met. I never wanted to see him again, but he persisted. He brought me flowers, called all the time, and showed up at Craig's house every Thursday night, whether I wanted him to or not. He even took care of me after I was "roofied" while on a revenge date. There was definitely something in that glass of wine. It was a date with a guy from school. He "seemed" so harmless. But like I said, he was persistent. And he did have a certain charm to him. I loved the way his mouth puckered, so I decided to give him another chance.

We went out again. Then I was the one coming over to his

house. First the lights went on, and then they went off. He made me feel like a queen. He was special. I loved being with him. We spent as much time as we could together for months.

I tried to get a job after graduation. The only thing I kept hearing was that the advertising world was not a place for women. At my first job interview, the guy who interviewed me actually told me to my face that he wouldn't hire me because I was too pretty. He said the men in his office wouldn't get any work done, because they would all be staring at me. He handed me back my resume and showed me to the door.

My second interview was worse. The guy interviewing me was a man who Rob had set me up to meet. We were just dating at the time, and this man was from a large, reputable advertising firm. Rob's company had used them. He looked at me and told me that models were interviewing at another desk. When I told him who I was, he just laughed. Said, "Good for Rob." Then told me he had never met a smart girl who looked like me before, and followed with "You would have a better chance at the modeling position." He handed me back my resume and walked away. This was when I was convinced that men were slime—and that I was really hot.

I had one more interview that week. This interview was with a small company in San Jose. There were three people in my first interview. One of the head guys in the firm was a teacher at San Jose State. He knew me well. He knew how hard I worked and what I had to offer. I thought I was a shoe-in. They hired one of the other people in my class. Someone who didn't get the grades I did, but then, he was a GUY!

Six interviews later I couldn't stand it anymore. I hated feeling like nothing I could do would matter. I gave up hope for an advertising career. I needed to make money. I saw an ad in the paper that American Airlines was looking for flight attendants. I knew I could do that. The advertising guys practically told me I could get a job like that by just showing up. I applied and within three weeks, I was living in Dallas going through training. Advertising guys are smart! Within three months, I was a full-fledged flight attendant. "Hi! I'm Sandi, fly me."

They told us when we signed up that we would have our choice of where we'd be stationed when we graduated. I could go back to San Francisco. This would be great. Rob and I could live happily ever after. What they didn't tell us was that our choice was their choice. San Francisco was not one of them. Neither was any other station anyone wanted to go to. We were all staying in Dallas, except a few who went to New York. I could have gone, but didn't want to be any further away from Rob.

They changed our looks. Showed us how they wanted us to wear our makeup. How to do our hair. They sent me to their hairdresser. He was having a bad day, hated women, or wasn't the genius they thought he would be. The idiot cut my hair short. Then said I looked hideous in short hair, so he bleached it blonde. He should have asked me before he did it. I knew short hair wasn't going to look good on me, I have a dozen photos of me with a pixie cut when I was five. Enough said!

Haircut and all, I loved the job—for a while. I was a first-class flight attendant replacement because I graduated top in my class. I had a whole bunch of "Thank You" cards, which were cards that American Airlines printed out and sent to their frequent fliers. If you were lucky enough to be flying with one of the passengers who had one of those cards, and they gave one to you, it was good for a one-way ticket anywhere American flew. FREE! I earned twenty-eight round-trip tickets in my first month. I'm such a slut. I used those tickets to go home to see Rob, travel to Hawaii (with Rob), meet Rob in San Francisco; it was great.

After the first year, I began to get sick on every flight I took. I would end up in the lavatory (bathroom) on almost every take-off and landing, which didn't instill a lot of confidence in the passengers. I liked to call it the "bile-high club." Then I had to work over the holidays. Then I began losing my balance. I remember on one particular flight, there was no turbulence or anything, but I was just so wobbly that I actually fell into a passenger's lap. The man was so nice about it. He just looked up, smiled, and said, "There is a God!" Then he handed me a "Thank You" card and a barf bag.

I was so embarrassed, but I felt okay because he made light of it. But I began to hate the job. I really hated it. I wanted to come home. Rob knew how sick I was and asked me to come home. He even mentioned the 'M' word. You know, Maalox. That was all it took. I quit, packed up everything, and moved home just in time for Christmas. I was so excited. I totally expected a ring for Christmas. I was going to get married.

I got myself all worked up and ready, and told all my friends and family. Then Christmas came, and instead of getting a ring, I got a pair of skis. What was he thinking? Sure they sparkled, but they didn't fit on my finger! I was so depressed. Was he not going to marry me now that I was back?

Valentine's Day came. I had one more shot. If not now, then I was going to give up. We sat in a restaurant, which would normally be a romantic restaurant with dim lighting. But they had just added a room that was as bright as the afternoon sun with not a cloud in the sky. There were children crying in the background, and a woman was staring at us as though she was expecting something to happen. And it did. Rob seemed to be waiting for just the right moment, but finally he just handed me a box and said, "Here, I was hoping for this to be a little more romantic, but . . ." In the box was a diamond. Not in a ring. Just a diamond. He wanted me to have it set the way I wanted. So I planned on having it set right next to a bigger diamond. And yes, I would marry him.

We got married in the gazebo at the Hyatt in San Jose. Rob didn't want a church wedding. We wanted a small get-together, but because we were both born and raised in the Bay Area, it ended up being a little larger than we anticipated. There were some two hundred and forty people at our wedding. We invited forty. Our parents had a field day. You would have thought they were the ones getting married. We didn't even know sixty percent of the people there. But we had fun.

After the festivities, we went to San Francisco and stayed at the Miyako Hotel. It is a Japanese-style hotel with all the flair of a Japanese hotel in Japan, or so my husband told me. There was a huge Japanese-style tub in the bathroom, where I sat naked while he poured warm water over me and gave me a bath. That was just the beginning of our honeymoon night. And I will leave the rest to your imagination.

The next morning we got up and ate a leisurely breakfast, packed our bags, and headed off to the airport to our final destination: Hawaii. We had a house waiting for us on the far end of the island of Kauai.

Once in Hawaii, it was totally not what I expected. I had dreamt of guys in Hawaiian shirts bringing me fancy drinks at the beach and girls standing on the sides doing the hula, shielding us from the wind and bringing us fresh fruit when they weren't dancing. Everyone would be smiling and greeting us as we passed, "Good morning, Mr. and Mrs. Selvi. Mrs. Selvi, would you be wanting a massage today?"

But my husband rented us a house all the way at the end of the island, right next to a farm. A chicken farm. There were no guys serving drinks, no girls giving us leis, no room-service, no pool, and definitely no massages. And a chicken farm meant roosters crowing at 5 a.m.: cock-a-doodle-doo, cock-a-doodle-doo! Those little fuckers woke me up just in time to see all the lizards crawling on the walls. I know they call them geckos, but "gecko" sounds cute. These were lizards. Hundreds of them were stuck against the wall with their skinny forked tongues sticking out at me. Why didn't anyone warn me? How did they get in? More importantly, how was I going to get them out?

Scream! That'll work. But screaming didn't get the lizards

out; it didn't get the two-inch spider off my T-shirt either. So here's how *that one* went...

We decided to go on a hike. Did I say we? Because I am almost positive I would never make the decision to do anything that resembled athletic behavior on a vacation. Especially on my honeymoon, except for sex, which, if you do it properly, can burn calories. A thirty-minute session of sex burns about 150 calories. An article I read on www.ezinearticles.com stated that you burn more calories with sex than: housework (111 calories), yoga (114 calories), or dancing (129 calories). Sex was how I had planned on getting my workouts. Not hiking!

Yes, my new husband, and now on the short list of almost ex-husbands, decided to take me for a hike. Have I mentioned I hate hiking? People weren't meant to hike. This is why God invented Jeeps.

We began our hike on a wide trail; the sun was shining. It was a beautiful day. As soon as we began to get a good stride going, the trail began to narrow and the sun disappeared. Rain began pouring down, and the trail became slippery. After my second slip, I didn't take my eyes off the trail. I was so fixated on the ground that I did not notice the tree that had fallen across the path in front of me. It was leaning against the hill. Still looking down I hit it head first. It knocked me back about two feet and almost knocked me out. But I wasn't going to give up. So onward I went, walking right into a spider's web. I didn't know what all that sticky stuff on my arms was. But I found out real quickly when I looked down, and right in the middle of my chest lay a spider that was larger than a silver dollar. After screaming and then dancing around trying to get the spider off, I sat and cried. The only thing I hate more than hiking: SPIDERS!

Rob wanted to make it up to me, so he surprised me the next day with a sunset helicopter ride. The ride began with Rob and me, and another couple, flying to an open space at the top of an inactive volcano. There Bob the pilot, spread out a blanket, poured champagne (one 7 Up for me), and set out some bread, cheese, and fruit. We had a few minutes to enjoy the view and then he was going to take us for a ride.

Bob, the psycho ex-Vietnam helicopter pilot, took us straight from there to the Na Pali coast. We were skimming the tops of the trees; I swear you could reach out and touch them. We went from the center of the island, and all you could see for miles was green. Through our headphones Bob piped in music. On came "Chariots of Fire" so loudly that you couldn't hear yourself think. We were flying so low and so fast. Ta ta ta da da. Ta ta da da da. TA TA TA DA DA. TA TAAAAAAA.

Then, all of a sudden, the music went dead, the helicopter slowed, I looked down, and we were over the edge. We were looking straight down a 4,000-foot cliff to the water. It was like having the floor dropped out from under you. And when I went to catch my breath, all I got was the stink of the guy sitting next to me. Not my soon-to-be-ex, but the husband of the other gal flying in the helicopter with us. He was wearing half a bottle of Ralph Lauren Polo. Up until that point, I actually liked that cologne. And yes, the helicopter had barf bags! Six to be exact.

I seriously believe that these unfortunate experiences on my honeymoon were caused by my lack of equilibrium. These were just a few more signs of M.S. in its early stages.

When we arrived home, I wanted to tell my parents all about my tragedies. I wanted them to feel the pain of my honeymoon as I had. I called up my mother and told her to put Dad on the other line. She told me that my father had left her. He waited until the day after I got married, and then he left. We all knew that my parents had been having troubles, but nothing like this. I was in total shock. Here I was embarking on a new life and new experience, and my parents' life together was over. I was confused and had no idea what to make of it. Then I kept thinking, "This is what's going to happen to me." I was scared, but I was also in love. I decided that I wasn't going to let it happen to me.

Rob and I were still living in his parents' duplex next door to our matchmaker, Craig. We had been looking for a house, but had no luck. Silicon Valley was very expensive, and we needed a lot more money for a down payment.

We had driven down a street that Rob had said he'd always liked because everyone on the street took such great care of their homes. He said he would love to buy a place there someday. Several months later, while we were on our way back from water-skiing—ski boat in tow—we saw a For Sale sign on the street he liked. He made a U-turn, which was pretty impressive with the boat, and we had ourselves a look.

We both fell in love. It was such an awesome house, with its yellow stone front matching the paint. It was a one-level, three-bedroom, two-and-a-half bath home, with a pond in the backyard. What wasn't there to love?

We talked to the agent, and she said we were almost $40,000 short. So we walked away—at least for the moment. We were going to try to figure out a way to come up with the money. Rob was going to work hard and something would come to him. I was going to dream, which I did. The lottery had just come out in California, and I decided maybe I could win the money. So I went to Longs Drugs on Bascom Avenue in Campbell and purchased one ticket. The ticket was a winner. I won two dollars. I thought if I kept doing that, eventually, after twenty thousand times, we would have the money.

So I asked the girl for my winnings. She asked if I wanted it in cash or two more tickets. I said, "Two more tickets, but make sure you give me a big winner; I'm trying to buy a house." I took my two tickets and my bag of supplies from Longs, got in my car, and began to drive the half a block to the duplex. When I hit the red light, I pulled out the tickets to scratch them off. The first one was Jokers Wild. It said at the top Match three like amounts and win that amount. Match two like amounts with a joker, and win double the amount. So I scratched the first amount, which was

$25,000. The second thing was a joker. Then a $2, then $5, then another $25,000. Did I read it wrong? Because I still had one more space to scratch, and if I read it right, I just won $50,000.

I kept looking at it and almost hit the car in front of me. Wasn't that girl sweet? Sometimes you got to know what to ask for. I called Rob right away.

"I won the lottery!" I yelled.

"I'm sorry, I'm working right now and can't talk to you," he replied.

"I won the lottery, and all you want to do is work?"

"Babe, I'm in a meeting," he said very angrily.

CLICK. He hung up on me.

His reaction came out of nowhere. I wanted him to be as excited as me, but he was acting like he was on a secret mission and didn't want to be disturbed. Either that or he was having an affair and didn't want to be disturbed. So I went next door, got Craig, and made him come over and look at the ticket. We called Rob back.

"I swear to God, I won the lottery, and don't you dare hang up on me again. Listen, here is Craig. He just came over, and I showed him the ticket."

"Oh my God! I can't believe this! She really won!" Craig said with such excitement.

I grabbed the phone. "So are you going to ignore me now? If so, I'll use the money to get me a Porsche, or how about a fur coat?"

"That's great, but I'm in a meeting. I'll be home around five o'clock. Can we talk about it then?"

"It's fucking Sunday. Can't you come home now so we can celebrate?" I begged. What I didn't realize at the time was that he was working hard to be successful, in a very stressful and competative field.

"Got to go," he said quietly. Then with a thundering sound, I could hear the phone CLICK. I was pissed. I wanted him to be as excited as I was, but he fell into his "business guy" mode and said, "do you know how much we are going to have to pay in taxes?" On the bright side he broke out the champagne and 7-up, then pointed out that we could now afford the house we both wanted.

I called the lottery office to see when they opened the next day so I could be the first one in line to cash my ticket. The recording said that the doors opened at 9:00 a.m.

I walked through the door at 9:01 a.m. I was shocked at the number of people cashing in their winning tickets already. It seemed like alot of people were there considering the short amount of time the lottery had been going on. The lottery had only started in California earlier that month. But the shock of seeing all the winners wore off quickly when I heard them talking.

Everyone was looking at each other's tickets, congratulating each other and laughing. Some had won $5. One person said they won $50. Another said he won $100, but I never heard any other amount larger than that. I didn't say a word. I stared straight ahead and stayed to myself. When I finally reached the girl at the front, she asked to see my ticket. I gave it to her. She looked at it, gave it a second look, and then screamed.

I was obviously the first big winner in our area. But did she have to yell out "$50, 000" over a ten-second time span? It got the attention of everyone in the room, everyone in the building, and everyone across the street. Everyone crowded around to see the person who had just handed in the $50,000 ticket, as if I did not stand out amongst the crowd already, being the only woman in the room. I felt like Charlie holding the golden ticket. I now had people touching me asking for my luck. Some, I think, were just touching me. Then some asked me for money. And yes, I was asked for my hand in marriage in seven languages. I just kept holding out my hand with the wedding ring on it, hopefully showing them all that I was already married. But this didn't stop the endless offers. I was told that Uncle Sam would take his share, and the rest would be sent via mail within three weeks. $40,000. Just what we needed.

Rob and I took the "promise to pay" from the lottery office, plus a huge chunk of change he had set aside for when we were ready to make an offer on the house. We got it. I gave the girl from Longs a bouquet of flowers.

Chapter 5
So, Miracles Happen?

There was a line of people waiting to stick their hands inside of me to see how far I was dilated. The first nurse was so animated, saying, "Hi Mrs. Selvi. How are you, Mrs. Selvi?" as she slipped on her glove. Then she stuck two fingers in. "Two centimeters, you're doing great! Can I get you some ice chips, some drugs, or maybe I can fluff your pillow?" She just stood there with a huge smile on her face. I wanted to smack her. Then an intern showed up already gloved. I didn't like him either. He reached in, taking what seemed to be a longer time than necessary, and then exclaimed, "You're getting close! You're about four centimeters." Next, a guy stuck his fingers in and yelled to the woman in the next room, "Hey babe. She's got you beat!" Then the last guy dropped the mop, stuck his hand inside, and yelled, "Si, she's ready!" It was at about this point that I began to think that some of these guys might not be doctors.

A year and a half after I was blissfully married, I ended up pregnant. We had talked about having children for a while; I had even gone off birth control pills. But I had been on the Pill for such a long time, I was afraid I might not get pregnant right away. I wondered how long that stuff stays in your system. If we were still counting, this could very well be theory #15 of why I think I have M.S.: birth control pills. Maybe they messed with my immune system?

My doctor had just given us the clearance to go ahead and try getting pregnant. He felt I had been off the Pill long enough to not hurt my chances of getting pregnant and not affect the baby. It worked on our first try. Sure, we had a lot of practice, but this was the big test. The funny thing was, I was never very good at taking tests. I always froze and couldn't remember what I was supposed to do. But wouldn't you know, the pregnancy test and drug tests were about the only tests I could do with my eyes closed and come up with big screaming positives, passing them with flying colors. Yeah, I knew I was pregnant on the first try. Rob thought I was insane and told me so. But I knew.

I went to the doctor and told him, "I know I'm pregnant." I knew it had only been a few weeks, but I was sure I was pregnant. I also told him that if I *was* pregnant to bill the insurance company; if I wasn't pregnant, I would come in and pay cash and never tell Rob that I even took the test. If I wasn't pregnant, I knew Rob would think I was even more insane than he already thought.

That afternoon, my doctor called and said, "Hey there. Well, I billed it to the insurance." And that was how I found out I was pregnant with my first son, the heir to the Selvi fortune.

Rob was in Chicago at the time, so I called to tell him. He knew. The first words out of his mouth were, "You're pregnant, aren't you?" He totally took the wind out of my sails. But it was the first time I ever had a reason to call him while he was away on business. He's a smart man.

It was an interesting pregnancy. I had a few complications, such as kidney infections, bladder infections, the usual fatigue, and my in-laws showing up. They had this habit of showing up at my door, unannounced, a few times a week, bearing gifts of fruit or baked goods. My husband kept telling me that they were trying to be nice. I kept telling him I wasn't used to that, and they were trying to kill me with carbs.

I'll never forget the time I was sunbathing topless. My doctor told me that once the baby was born, breast-feeding was going to hurt. He said if you toughen your nipples by exposing them to the sun, it helps. So there I was, sunbathing in the backyard, *my* backyard, when all of a sudden my in-laws came around the corner, calling cheerfully, "Hi, honey!"

I could have just died.

But I had a reprieve. Rob came home and told me that he was being transferred to France. We would be moving over there right after the baby was born and staying there for two years, just my husband, the baby, and me. No in-laws. Wait—that means no my mom either, or no friends!

I went into labor, and Jim was born approximately twelve hours later. I went into labor while Rob was on a business trip to Sonoma. I called him and told him that I was heading to the hospital. He drove straight back from his off-site meeting to join me there. My mother drove me to the hospital and filled in until he arrived. I kept asking her questions about labor and delivery only to hear that she had no idea because both my brother and I were born Caesarean.

I didn't want any drugs. I wanted to do this as naturally as I could. Everyone was so nice and sweet, and so was I when the whole thing started. The nurses checked me in and put me in my bed. They strapped me to all the monitors, and there I stayed. The phone rang every fifteen minutes. It was Rob. He was giving me blow-by-blow details of his 90 to 100 M.P.H. driving escapade from Sonoma. I told him to slow down. He said, "How many times do you think I'll ever get to use this line: My wife is having a BABY! And mean it?"

Rob finally arrived at the hospital. In one way, I was happy to see him; in other ways, I just wanted to hurt him. The pain I was now feeling from the contractions was getting uncomfortable. Happy Sandi must have stepped outside for a break. He came over, kissed me, and began rubbing my shoulders. I told him he was not allowed to touch me. EVER AGAIN. *He* did this to me. He was the reason I was in so much pain. The nurse told him to rub my back. She basically began to tell him what to do, and he did it. She was the nurse from hell. She made Nurse Ratchet look like a saint. I loved her.

The contractions began to get worse. Not only that, when there weren't contractions, there was this person inside of me kicking to get out—kicking! Kicking my ribs, my bladder, and occasionally, my brain, reminding me how I got this way, which I would then get angry about and tell my husband to go away and leave me alone. Touching me was not an option anymore, and if he had tried to kiss me, I would have either bit off his lip or tongue because I knew where kissing led. And that was never going to happen again. NEVER!

The pain was tremendous. There was no more counting the time between the contractions. It was just one big contraction. The line of people waiting to stick their fingers up inside me had dissipated. Then the doctor came in and conferred with the last guy, and told me it was indeed time. That was when I began to push with all my might, trying to free myself of this pain. But nothing was happening. I was too tired. I had nothing left. "Let's forget about it for today," I begged. But the nurses begged me to push, the doctor begged me to push, and even Rob begged me to push. Nope! I had nothing left. Then the doctor picked up the forceps and gave them a loud CLANK. "I'm going to have to use the forceps." I took one look at them, remembering my friend Lisa with that weird scar on her forehead, and remembering her mother's sweet little voice, "Well, she's always been a little stubborn. Even the day she was born, she had to be pulled out with forceps." That was where I had heard that word before.

"That's why my poor little Lisa has that scar on her forehead. Poor dear, scarred for life." She sounded so sad when she said that.

Scarred for life. Scarred for life? I pushed so hard and so fast that the baby flew out.

Then the doctor yelled, "Stop pushing now."

"Put the forceps down, and I'll stop pushing," I replied.

Gently he said, "Mrs. Selvi, please stop pushing. The cord is wrapped around his neck."

"His?" I stopped pushing. "It's a boy?"

He unwrapped the cord from Jim's neck, and Jim screamed.

Jim. That was his name, we had already decided. If it was boy, his name would be Jim. *James Robert.* Jim Bob.

"Yes, a perfect baby boy."

Then he handed the scissors to my husband and said, "Would you like to cut the cord?"

The only thing Rob could say was, "Isn't there anyone here a little more qualified?"

"Si. I cut da cord," came a voice as we heard the mop hit the floor again.

After Jim was born, Rob went to France ahead of me. He had to get things straightened out in France, while I stayed in California with my mother and got used to being a mom. Rob had already started working, so he needed to get back and get used to a new culture.

He bought a bed, some towels, and a few other things to get by until everything, including me and the baby, arrived from America. Our things had all been sent by boat and we were hoping they would arrive the same week I did. That was the plan.

Rob called to tell me that he had also bought a car, a small get-around car—a 'Deux Cheveaux,' which was a paper-thin, two-ounce car, with an engine that could barely get up our driveway (let alone a hill). *Deux Cheveaux,* translation: "two horses." Yep, that was about all the horsepower that little car had, but it smelled like three.

Living in France was a trip. It was so different from living in the United States, especially because I didn't know a single word of French when I first found out I would be living there. You soon understand that if you don't speak the language, you won't survive. I learned that from my grandparents and my father. My father still complains about not knowing English until he went in to kindergarten. They only spoke Italian at home. Sink or swim, he told me. He learned English very quickly; he swam. I learned to swim very quickly too.

In the village next to ours, we had an outdoor market. You

could go to the individual stands to purchase your vegetables and fruits. You were never allowed to touch the items, but you could ask for what you wanted. Easy if you spoke the language. The one stand I enjoyed the most, which had the freshest produce, was owned by a man who was incorrigible. This man insisted I order my veggies in perfect French, or he wouldn't sell them to me, he would completely ignore me. I would get out my dictionary, look up the vegetable I wanted, then slaughtered it. Nine times out of ten I was right, but that one time he would stop me. He demanded that I repeat after him. He acted as if he couldn't understand me when I spoke English. In his smug way he would say things like *"Non, madame. Répétition après moi. Trois pommes de terre s'il vous plaît."*

I did it. I repeated after him, and he would laugh and make me do it again. I felt like an idiot, but it worked. After two months, I was speaking perfect produce French.

That's when he looked me in the eye, and in perfect English said, "Madame, your French is perfect. If I did not know better, I would think you were from this beautiful nation."

"You speak English?" I demanded.

"But of course," he said smugly.

"Fuck you! There's some French you didn't need to teach me."

I walked away thinking how he had tortured me. *Répétition après moi.* "I hate the French!" Other than the French, living in France was magical. My husband and I really enjoyed each other and our new son, Jim. We (Jim and I) went to every museum. We spent more time on the RER (Réseau Express Régional, or also known as the subway!) discovering Paris than sitting at home. There were no outside influences to bother us, we just had fun. We spent quality time with each other. But that ended too soon. Rob finished a job that was supposed to last two years in only a year and two months. We stayed in France for a little longer, traveling and having fun. Then it was back to the States.

We moved back in December of 1988. I came home a few days earlier than Rob, because he had to finish up a few last-minute things at the office. He would be home just in time for Christmas. Then he called me and said that Lou, his best friend from college, had been in Germany again. They'd made arrangements to meet in England. He was going to fly into New York with Lou, then fly home to San Francisco from there. He thought it would be more fun to travel with his friend and have someone to talk to on the long journey home.

Earlier on, Lou had been in France to visit us. He worked for Volkswagen and was on his way back to the United States to see his family too. He and his wife, Maria, had just recently had another child. They already had two children who were a lot older (Rob is the older son's godfather), but family meant so much to them that they decided to have a second family. Having him on the plane would be great for Rob. I knew that Lou was fun, so I thought, "Good, he'll keep Rob company." He was such a great guy. I was glad he and Rob were going to get to spend more time together.

I was at the house, wrapping presents and decorating the tree, when Lou's wife Maria called. She needed to talk to Rob. I told her that Rob was on his way home from France. Then I told her that Rob had just called the day before; he and Lou were meeting in London and flying home together. Dead silence followed. I knew something was really wrong. When Maria finally spoke, she sounded so upset. She told me that she had gotten a call from Pan Am, and that Lou was on flight 103, the flight that blew up over Lockerbee, Scotland. Rob was their executor, the one Lou told Maria to call if anything ever happened to him. She wanted help. She was hoping Rob wasn't with Lou. So was I.

I turned on the news. The incident was all they covered. I got on the phone and began calling everyone trying to find out if Rob had actually gotten on that flight.

No one would tell me anything. I called Pan Am, and then

I called American Airlines, which was the airlines he was booked with before he changed his plans. Nobody was talking. Nobody knew where he was.

I watched the plane blow up, over and over again on TV. It was the only thing on TV. I walked the floor, pacing up and down, not saying a word. My mother just held our son and watched me pace. I knew he was still alive. I would hear from him.

Three hours later. Nothing.

Five hours later. Nothing.

Maria called again. She had just heard from Pan Am again, confirming that Lou had definitely been on the plane. I still hadn't heard from Rob, and Pan Am hadn't called me.

Nothing. I still paced the floors some more. Every few minutes I kissed my son. My mother hugged me. We never said a word. Six hours after the crash, the phone rang. It was Maria again. They had just confirmed that another friend of theirs had been on the plane too; he'd been sitting next to Lou. She wanted to know if I had heard from anyone yet. Nearly an hour later, seven hours after the plane blew up, the phone rang again. My heart was beating out of my chest. I prayed that it was not Pan Am.

"Hey babe, just got off the flight, Chuck (his best friend) picked me up from the airport." That's all I heard before I began crying. Yes, it was Rob. He was totally oblivious to what had happened. He was calling to tell me that he was going out for a drink with a friend, Chuck, and would be home later. I was crying so hard that I couldn't talk. But I could say, "Get your ass home."

He could barely understand me. My mother took the phone and explained what had happened. She explained what I had been thinking all day and hinted that he had better come home. When he arrived, I just held him for hours. He called Maria. It was so sad around our house. But inside I felt guilty, I was so thankful that Rob wasn't on that flight. So thankful that I got pregnant again, because that's how it happens, girls. We had talked about having a second one. We wanted them to be really close together. But I wasn't getting pregnant right away, and so we'd decided to wait. That wasn't in the cards. Love conquers all. I ended up pregnant.

This pregnancy was so much more difficult than the first. I was sick all the time. I had kidney infections and bladder infections again. I couldn't sleep, and was constantly tired. I was so exhausted, I couldn't get out of bed, night or day.

I went into labor prematurely, six weeks prematurely.

The doctors stopped it. Rob wasn't even in the United States at the time. He was in Mexico with one of his friends—his friend Jim, who we named our first child after. Big Jim had opened a bar in Cabo, and Rob wanted to be there for the grand opening. I was thrilled Rob could be there. It was only for a week, and I wasn't due for at least another month. Well, that was what we thought anyways.

So Rob had gone to Mexico, and I had gone into labor. I spent a few days in the hospital, and the doctors stopped the labor, just in time for me to be able to pick Rob up from the airport. On the day he returned, I showed up at the airport all excited to hear about the bar. On our way home, I felt a contraction, then another and another. We ended up driving straight to the hospital, checking in, and going into hard labor. The doctors determined that the baby was a little less than five weeks premature at this point, so they left me in labor. Hard labor. But they said it was best for the baby. I was okay with that.

Five days later, yes, FIVE days later, my second son, Tom, was born. I was so sick after Tom was born that I needed help. Rob was in and out of the hospital. My mother was there for a while, and then we hired a high school girl to come in and help. My back was trashed. I had ruptured two discs in my back during labor, and I needed surgery.

All of a sudden, I didn't feel the connection I had felt with my husband just months earlier. Now, I was feeling alone and useless. He was working more hours, finding reasons to be home less. And when Rob was home, he wasn't pleasant.

He always found something to complain about. Nothing was good enough. The house wasn't neat enough. The kids were too noisy. Dinner wasn't to his liking. So he worked even more. I needed help. I could hardly walk; I was exhausted. I couldn't please my husband no matter how hard I tried.

Then I would look in the mirror and hate myself. No wonder he didn't want to be with me. I looked horrible. When I was breast-feeding, I had big, wonderful breasts. Now, they looked like deflated balloons. I cried and told my husband that the old woman in the back of the *Playboy* looked better than me.

For Mother's Day that year, I got a card with the name of a plastic surgeon in it. How inventive of Hallmark. I went to see the surgeon, and he fixed me up. He put in breast implants, and I looked great. Then all the news came out about silicon implants. I always seem to be in the wrong place at the wrong time. I was scared. My body began to reject my implants. It built up a casing around the implants that became so hard that it was like having rocks in my chest. I have had love in my heart but never rocks in my chest. The implants hurt all the time.

After seeing the surgeon again, I was told the implants had to come out, but they could be replaced with the saline ones. Within two weeks, I had a new set of boobs.

But they didn't fix any of my problems.

I would hear Rob's car coming down the street and begin to shake. I would run around the house to make sure everything was in its place and things were perfect, so that I didn't have to hear his complaints. It didn't matter; if there was one piece of paper on the floor, he would find it, and I would hear about it. My back was getting worse, and I was feeling horrible.

I had my first back surgery almost two years to the date after my son was born. Then one day Rob found three different pill bottles from three different doctors. I was popping painkillers like they were candy. He took me into the Spine Center Institute in Daly City, where they had me signed, sealed, and prepared for surgery before Christmas. We hired a young high school girl to help out. A few days after my surgery, the high school girl we hired to take care of the boys spilled milk on the floor.

It was a white floor.

I didn't see it.

I slipped and fell. And I thought needles hurt. This felt like five hundred needles—all at the same time.

Never trust a high school girl. I needed a second surgery, but I wanted to wait.

We moved to Saratoga right before my second back surgery; it was almost a year to the day later when I hired a live-in nanny. She was a young girl from Switzerland. Her cousin worked for a friend of my husband's in Saratoga. She lived with us and basically took Rob's place. She became my friend and confidant. Rob was never home. I know he was focusing on his career, but I kept thinking that he was probably out with a high school girl.

After my second back surgery, I began to feel a little stronger. Rob and I were getting along much better, because I was taking care of myself. I learned early that I needed to take care of me and all else would follow. I was doing tae kwon do to help improve my strength and balance, and I was even teaching classes two days a week. I had gone from a white belt to a red belt in a little over four years. I was also volunteering at the kids' school and teaching Sunday school at the church. I was coaching soccer and basketball.

I thought things were going great. That was when I fell trying to do that spin kick. That was when my life began to spin out of control. Everything that happened from that day forward is what made me take a chance at something, anything, to change my downward trajectory. I was happy I had that option and the cash.

Chapter 6
Stem Cell Indictment

Even though I was told I was going to be asked by Diane Feinstein to speak to congress, the call never came. They didn't need me once Barack Obama became president. But if I had gone, I knew exactly what I was going to say...

> *"Hey! Dumb Shits, stop mixing religion and politics. As you can see in the Middle East and throughout history, politics and religion don't mix. How many times did you go to a party when you were young and the last thing your father told you as you left the house, 'Don't talk about religion or Politics.' Even my father, who was a cop, knew back when I was a child if you mix those subjects, be ready to call in SWAT, and even then nobody wins. As you can see, Stem Cell Transplants do work, I am living proof. Thank You for your time."*

So, that is what I would have said, if given the chance!

There are four types of stem cell transplants:

* Embryonic stem cells, taken from human embryos
* Fetal stem cells, taken from aborted fetal tissue
* Umbilical stem cells, taken from umbilical cords
* Adult stem cells, taken from adult tissue

Embryonic stem cells are formed during the early stages of embryonic development, which remain undifferentiated and have the ability to become, or differentiate, into almost any tissue in the body. They are the stem cells of life. For example, you can take cells from one section of an embryo, that might have become part of the liver, and transfer them into another section of the embryo, where they can now develop into muscle, nerve, or blood cells. The amazing thing is that anyone could accept these cells with no problems of rejection because the embryo has not yet developed enough to be recognized as a separate individual with its own DNA.

During the Bush administration, thousands of embryos were thrown out every day— wasted, because President George W. Bush had "religious issues" with this area of science. I repeat, SCIENCE. He did not want to mess with God. He did not want the frozen embryos going to stem cell research.

Excuse me, Dub'ya, but you're throwing away "in vitro cells" that *could* possibly grow one day into a human if you thaw them out properly. And you're worried that you might cross the line with God over saving lives? Bastard! Throwing away stem cells that could be put to good use. At least give what was going to be thrown away a chance to save a life. Personally, I believe that religion and politics don't mix. But that is just my opinion. And the turmoil in the Middle East only strengthens my belief. Religion and politics—really don't mix. Doesn't look like they ever have.

Anyway, when a woman goes in for in vitro fertilization, she has six to eight eggs extracted, and each egg is then fertilized. Only one or two eggs are implanted, and the others are frozen. If the parents of the eggs find out they've become pregnant, and don't want any more children, it is up to *them* to decide what they want to do with the remaining embryos. Not the government. If they want to donate their fertilized eggs to help another couple have a child, help a person suffering from a debilitating disease, or make an omelet, whatever, good for them.

If you take the cells from an embryo and transfer them into a Petri dish, they can be grown indefinitely. These are known as "embryonic stem cell lines." Taking the embryos they throw out from one clinic in one day, we would never have to harvest stem cells again in the United States. Ever.

Fetal stem cells are extracted from the fetus after it has been aborted. Thank God we still have the right to choose. This is what most of the uproar is all about. These cells, like embryonic stem cells, can morph into many different types of cells. But the cells come from a fetus. These cells can be rejected because the fetus has begun to develop its own DNA. In most cases, the cells are useful and helpful. If an embryo is going to be aborted, can't we give it a purpose?

Umbilical cord blood is especially rich in stem cells that give rise to red blood cells and lymphocytes. Some parents choose to save the cord blood in private cord blood banks. It can be used later, if needed, as an alternative use to a bone marrow transplant. Studies have shown that people not related to the donor (genetically mismatched) can benefit from transplants of umbilical cord blood in combating leukemia and other cancers. Cord blood has also been used to repair heart and other tissue defects in children with certain metabolic disorders.

Adult stem cells are generally found in the bone marrow, but have recently been found in fat tissue removed through liposuction. They can usually only help the donor. In some cases, family members can use each other's stem cells. Rarely can someone use a donor's cells without having to take anti-rejection medication.

I had an autologous transplant, which used my own adult stem cells. People don't hear much about this type of transplant because it gets lost in all the glory and uproar of embryonic stem cell research. What bothers me is the fact that people still refer to them as fetal stem cells, which causes such a stir. But what I'm gathering from my own research, and my own reality, is that an autologous transplant can do just as much good. Just look at me.

This is how it was supposed to go: first, they were going to put a Mediport in my chest through a main artery. Then they were going to take my own stem cells out through a different machine that would work with the Mediport. The machine would funnel my blood at a high rate of speed, separating the stem cells from the blood. The stem cells would then be cleaned up and frozen. Radiation and chemotherapy would follow. Afterwards, they would be able to give me back my stem cells. They said that theoretically, my M.S. should come to a stop, and possibly, I could get better. My body would no longer be fighting itself, so it would have time to heal. Oh, and by the way, most insurance plans won't cover a penny.

When I was first diagnosed with M.S., my MRI showed six lesions, which seemed to alarm my doctor. My next MRI showed quite a few more. One time, while stuck waiting in the doctor's office, I pulled out my MRI, which is like basically twenty x-rays of your brain, each film representing a different layer. If you hold them up to the light, the films show that your brain is gray, with an elongated X in the center, where the spinal cord enters the brain. You can see that the natural folds in the brain are outlined in a lighter gray, and the skull is obvious because it's dark, almost black, with a thin line of white surrounding it. The brain is supposed to be pretty even in color, but with M.S., you see random white spots that are scattered amidst the gray, making the MRI image look like a Jackson Pollock painting.

I personally counted eighteen white spots on my MRI. But I am no *specialist*. Without the doctor even telling me, I knew I was progressing rapidly. I wanted the transplant. The doctors warned me that some people had died from the procedure, but I thought, living with M.S. or dying, which could be worse? And yes, I was scared. I thought of nothing else for weeks. I wanted to be better or be dead, it was as simple as that. After seeing all the people at the National Multiple Sclerosis Society, I decided I didn't want to be taken care of for the rest of my life. I didn't like where I was headed. Hell, I didn't *know* where I was headed, but I knew it wasn't good. But I did like the idea that something out there might be able to help me, and possibly others just like me. I was willing to take the chance to see.

After two months of tests, tests, and more tests, I was approved, which meant I had to leave my two boys, and all my friends, live down in San Diego for at least two months, and pray. Did I say "pray"? I meant "pay." Rob and I rented the cutest little house right down the block from the beach, a few minutes from the hospital in La Jolla. Nothing special. But it was clean and I had my own room. We had separate rooms, because I didn't want to wake him up—I knew it would be difficult to sleep during this process. We knew it would all work out.

I turned forty on March 15, 2000. March 16th, I had the Mediport put in my chest. It was great in theory. But when it comes right down to it, when they put the port in, they punctured my lung. Shit happens.

I told the nurse that I couldn't breathe, and she gave me Ativan, also known by the name Lorazepam. It's a powerful anxiolytic, and since its introduction in 1977, its principal use has been treating the symptom of anxiety. It calms you down. She thought I was panicking. An hour later, when I told her I was really scared because I still couldn't breathe, she gave me two more doses of Ativan and sent me home. I have to say, the shit works. It took all the anxiety out of me thinking I was dying. I spent all night propped up, coughing and listening to a tape of Brian Regan (which was one of the comedy tapes I bought at Costco while getting supplies for my procedure). I was afraid to fall asleep. I couldn't breathe. I think the only reason why I didn't die that night was because I was laughing between the coughs.

When we returned to the hospital in the morning, they rushed me in for surgery to refill my lung. They used something called a Heimlich valve, after its inventor, Henry Heimlich. It is a one-way valve used in respiratory medicine to prevent air from traveling back. As soon as it was in place, the pain in my chest immediately went away.

My son Jim, who was ten years old at the time, arrived the next day. It was his first solo flight, no parents, no brother. Just him. Our younger son, Tom, was too scared to fly alone, so Jim arrived all happy because his brother couldn't come. Only one problem. Jim was beginning to get a cold. He had the sniffles. They wouldn't let him in to see me. I remember crying, so they let him see me heavily clad in a mask and gloves, and we were allowed fifteen minutes together. I couldn't see him the rest of the time he was in San Diego.

I was running a fever, from the Neupogen, which is the brand name for a filgrastim (a protein that stimulates the production of white blood cells). I had to have those Neupogen shots for days in preparation for the Pharisees, the machine used to separate stem cells from blood. So they kept me on antibiotics as a prophylactic. My fever kept spiking. Although they didn't keep me in the hospital, they told us if it got over 100.8 degrees, we had to call. We called a couple of times, and each time, they suggested Tylenol and said if that didn't work, I would have to come in. It worked.

Every time I went to the hospital, they took nine vials of blood, checking for anything and everything. Then we would go off to breakfast and then the Pharisees began. The Pharisees machine was a machine that funneled my blood out of one of the tubes in my chest and into the machine. The machine would then spin at such a rate that the stem cells would separate from my blood, pumping my blood back through the other tube. I would sit for hours at a time, with my computer in hand, writing. I had always told my kids stories at night to help them fall asleep, and I wanted to write them down for them if I wasn't around to tell them later.

We knew my hair was going to be falling out at some point, so Rob had a great idea. He wanted to take me to a hair salon and have my hair cut short, so that when it did begin to fall out it wouldn't be such a shock. My hair had been at least shoulder length since I had that hideous haircut when I was a flight attendant and the pixie cut before that. I was nervous, but I did it and got the cutest haircut. I loved my new look, but it was a little dull; they cut off all my blond. Rob decided to make it fun, so he sat me on the patio of the rental house and bleached it for me. It really was cute.

The Pharisees took several days to collect the millions of stem cells needed to carry on with the procedure. Afterward, I needed to be mapped for radiation. They stuck me on a cold metal table, took x-rays, and dotted me with permanent little blue tattoos. Eight of them. Remember the scene in *Friends* where Phoebe goes to get a tattoo of her mother's name? She doesn't like the tattoo process after one prick, so she ends up with one blue dot the size of a small freckle. She explains that it was her mother's view of the Earth as she watched over her. That means I must have eight people watching over me. They are eight little pinpoint marks in blue. These blue tattoos are important: it's what they used to line me up in the machine for radiation. It's important that you are in the same place every time so that you don't   accidentally radiate something you shouldn't. They took measurements and made a lead plate especially built to cover the areas of the body that are sensitive to radiation. It went from the bottom of my chin to my pubic bone.

The preparation for the transplant was complete.

I was then sent out into the world for my last romp. I was told to go do whatever I wanted to do because as soon as the chemo began, I would be isolated. We went to the zoo. Rob got a wheelchair and pushed me from one end to the other. I ate a corn dog and had some cotton candy—my two most favorite comfort foods in the world. When we got home that afternoon my hair began falling out. It was so strange—no, it was the Neupogen. One of the side effects from Neupogen: hair loss. It was a little at first, and it itched like crazy. Then it began coming out by the handful. Freaky! And what little hair I did have left, itched so much. Rob finally just shaved my head. End of problem. But now I was cold all the time. That was what the hats were for; the ones Deb, the gal who went before me in the stem cell process, and her mother-in-law had dropped off the day before. I had no idea how much my hair had kept me warm. Deb knew!

Then there was chemo. What an ordeal. The nurses came into the room, dressed in lead aprons, with full head masks on and gloves up to their armpits. They looked like they were wearing hazmat gear. They were carrying a bag of gunk. They hooked it up to my I.V. and backed away. It was scary! For good reason too. I got so sick from it. First I couldn't stop throwing up. And then stuff was coming out of both ends at the same time. This is when things began to get messy. I felt so sorry for Rob for having to constantly clean up after me. As sick as I was, I couldn't do anything. But everything in the house had to be sterile. Which left him to do all the dirty work.

Every time we went to the hospital after chemo, they took blood and gave me I.V. solutions of all kinds, and massive amounts of potassium. One of the side effects of chemo is loss of potassium. The doctors told me that because I was throwing up so much (and the other thing), I became dehydrated. The potassium levels in my body had dropped dangerously low. They went on to explain how your body needs potassium; it's one of the main electrolytes, which is what maintains the electrical potential of the cell. This is especially important in cells with high electrical activity, such as nerves and muscles. The lack of potassium caused cramping in my muscles and tremors all over my body.

I had to report what I ate and drank, how much I peed and pooped, and which medications I had taken and when (sometimes on an hourly basis). My new friend Deb gave me this great solution for taking the meds. She suggested putting my medications in little plastic cups with lids on them. The cups were about two inches in diameter. We could put all my meds in these little containers and write the time and day to take them on the lid. It was so much simpler than having to open each bottle every hour.

The next thing on our agenda was radiation. Radiation didn't hurt. It was like taking a long x-ray. I was uncomfortable because the table was cold and hard, but it didn't hurt a bit. The first day was mapping, and the second day was full body radiation. This made me even sicker. Poor Rob had to take care of me, cook for me, and clean up my messes—again!

But he had to go back to Saratoga that week. I was looking forward to my mother coming down to stay with me, but this was when she began to get sick herself and didn't want to tell me, she had the first signs of Breast Cancer; eventually she had to tell me. It was a mad dash to find someone to take Rob's place, but two of my best friends stepped up. First Gayle would come, then Shelley. Both friends since our children were toddlers. My poor friends had no idea what they were getting themselves in to.

It was March 31—some sixteen days after having my lung punctured—that I became a new person. March 31, 2000, was the day I received my stem cells back. The experts call this ground zero. The stem cells came in a pouch, like the I.V. solutions and chemo, except they were orange. The stem cells were fed back to me through my port. And all for the small price of just under $100,000. (There goes the beach house.)

Every day following radiation, I reported back to the hospital. They would take more blood, feed me, and then give me more potassium. Some days I would spend four or five hours just receiving potassium. Thank God for the comedy tapes. I would have been bored out of my mind without them! I began listening to them day and night.

When my friend Gayle came to take over for Rob, we played cards and ate good food, which had to be prepared according to the hospital's standards (which meant meat had to be cooked at a certain temperature. and every can, bottle and utensil had to be sterilized before I could touch them). She took care of me. Cleaned up my messes, fed me food, and kicked my ass at cards.

My fever would spike all the time. I was so uncomfortable physically and emotionally that I would cry at the drop of a hat. The doctors were worried about my mental state, so they sent me to a psychiatrist. He said I was depressed. No shit! I hadn't seen my kids in over a month. I missed seeing my youngest son get his braces off. All I did was throw up (and I've already told you about the diarrhea). I was still sick as a dog, so they put me on antidepressants. There is one thing I have learned about antidepressants. They work if you have a chemical imbalance, but if your life truly sucks, they don't work at all. I was still depressed. So I listened to more comedy. I listened to John Pinette, Bobby Collins, and Pablo Francisco. As sick as I was, I managed to eke out a chuckle every once in a while.

They started giving me platelets. Yes, I had no platelets. Don't worry, I had no idea what that meant either. I had to look it up. Wikipedia says, Platelets: blah blah blah…play a fundamental role in hemostasis (I had to look that one up too) and are a natural source of growth factors. They circulate in the blood of mammals and are involved in hemostasis, leading to the formation of blood clots. Hemostasis: a complex process, which causes the bleeding process to stop. Without them you could bleed to death.

Apparently platelets are important and thank God they were giving them to me! Please sir…may I have some more? They were also giving me antibiotics, and of course, lots of potassium. They were telling me that the potassium was even more important now because it would help balance the platelets.

Shelley took Gayle's place. Gayle couldn't spend the entire two weeks with me, so she and Shelley split the time. What great friends I had to take the time out of their busy lives to be there for me. I am so blessed in so many ways.

Rob came back just in time to deal with the infected Mediport. Yes, the doctors and nurses decided that the reason my fever was now spiking was because my Mediport was infected and had to be removed. I was scared to death. The doctor patted me on the head, put one hand on my chest, and pulled the thing out. Sure, he used a little numbing medication—but it didn't work. I felt the thing come out. I almost passed out. But I was now free. I would never have to swab that thing again. Well, obviously I had not swabbed it well enough, otherwise it wouldn't have gotten infected in the first place. Either way, I was glad to be rid of it.

I kept thinking about when I had to go back to the hospital the next morning. How were they going to take my blood or give me potassium? An I.V.? I hate those things too.

My mom was well enough to come down for the last week. I was wearing diapers because I still had diarrhea and peed every time I stood up. On the way to the hospital, my mom popped the tire on my car by running into the curb: $231 for a tire. Shit happens. I don't think my first car cost $231. Wow, I should pay more attention to how much I'm paying for things. I seriously had no idea tires were so expensive. It was a Volkswagen Bug for God's sake.

By April 20th, twenty-one days after my transplant, I was feeling quite good. I had several excellent days. I was a little sad that I was going to miss Easter, but I had everything set up for Rob to deliver Easter baskets. And my Richard Belzer tape would keep me company. I remembered hearing him on the Howard Stern show. The tape would keep me company—he's hysterical! Still one of my favorites.

A week after Easter, it had been almost two months since I had seen my kids. Other than Jim's fifteen-minute visit at the beginning of my journey. That day, the day I arrived home, was the most special day I can remember since they were born. I was so excited to see them. Being away from them that long had to be the hardest thing I had ever done. The stem cell transplant seemed like a piece of cake compared to missing my boys.

I went down to San Diego once a month after that for checkups. Everything was going great. My new friend, Deb, and I talked frequently. We compared notes and bitched about the few remaining symptoms we each still had.

In November of that same year, I received a phone call saying that Deb was ill again. On my monthly visit to San Diego that bleak November, I went to see her. She passed away two days later—a little more than one year after her transplant. Even though they told me it had nothing to do with her transplant, I couldn't help but wonder. Was shit going to happen to me again? I was again angry, frustrated, and scared. No one could understand how I felt inside. I no longer had Deb to compare notes with, and worse, the world no longer had an angel. After all she had gone through (and boy, did I know!), to just die like that, it wasn't fair. She deserved so much better. She deserved a frickin' medal: "The Generous Heart." I sat around the house and cried for days. Rob didn't know what to do with me. I was so scared and confused.

Sure, my symptoms were going away slowly, but so had Deb's. I just kept waiting for my number to come up. Though one day in December, almost a month after Deb's death, I thought about it. My life had already completely changed. I was feeling better. It had been nine months since the transplant, and I didn't have the pain I used to have all the time. That was something. The transplant seemed to work. Then I began to think, "What if today were my last day?" and then I thought, "Why don't I treat each day as if it were?" Before my transplant, I was so careful and sad. But now, I had been listening to comedy, and I laughed all the time. I saw life in a different light. I was going to change my ways. I was going to try and laugh at everything, make it funny. I was going to have to look more closely at this thing called comedy.

I realized I no longer had double vision. I no longer needed a cane to walk, and my speech was no longer slurred or garbled. But there were many times I had small problems that made me think that the procedure hadn't worked (such as the numerous times I dropped my pen, or tripped over what I swear was the cat. Again, that's my story and I'm sticking to it). I remembered Deb. Then one afternoon I jumped out of bed, ran to the bathroom, looked in the mirror, and reminded myself that it wasn't that long ago I couldn't even walk. And now look, I just ran!

The procedure *did* work. I could travel again. I was getting better every day. It was hard for me to see because it happened in such small baby steps, but the baby steps were in the right direction—away from the wheelchair and further from the cemetery. My friends all noticed a difference.

Yes, I still have M.S. I have small reminders of it every day. I tend to still walk with a little limp. I have a little drop in my left foot—but not like I once did. My sensitivity to heat is not as bad as it once was, but I do not like to test it. I no longer walk with a cane. Flying on an airplane is okay again. My bladder control is back. Eventually the tremors went away, so I could write. And hold a cup of coffee without wearing it! This saved me hundreds of dollars in spilled lattes and dry cleaning. The writing thing, well, what do you think so far?

Chapter 7
I Can't Give Up?

We spent all day in the doctor's office. When we got in the car, all my mother said to me (in her deep, raspy voice) was, "I can't believe you told that doctor I smoked cigarettes." I said, "Well, Darth, I think he would've been able to tell when you tried to light the tongue depressor on fire. Or maybe he could tell from the cigarette pack rolled up in your sleeve."

I was feeling so much healthier after my transplant that when my mother became ill, I was able to take care of her. I loved my mother so much; it was such an honor to be there for her. I can honestly say she was my best friend. It was hard to see her go like she did.

My mom had been diagnosed with breast cancer, chronic obstructive pulmonary disease (COPD), and congestive heart failure, in that order. The breast cancer was first to arrive. What a blow. She went through radiation and took Tamoxifen, a drug that blocks the estrogen receptors on cancer cells and is used in the treatment of breast cancer).

No more cancer.

But the radiation dried out her lungs. Radiation and years of smoking, not a good combo. Her voice was the first thing to change. It had always been scratchy in a sexy kind of way, but it slowly worsened. Her speech was interrupted by a hacking cough every few minutes. Then her eyes lost their clarity, it was like a cloud was covering the blue of her eyes. Her chest swelled to grossly abnormal proportions. She had what the doctors called a "barrel chest," which is exactly what it looked like. Her body had puffed up two sizes larger than normal due to the prednisone they constantly pumped into her.

At that time my mother could no longer take care of herself, so she moved in with my family and me for three years before she died. She was on oxygen 24/7. We had an oxygen machine set up in the back room. She wore her over-the-ear nasal cannula (the oxygen tube that attaches under the nose), which was connected to an eighty-foot tube that she used when she wanted to come to the dinner table. It broke my heart to see her looking so unhealthy because she had always been this cute little thing everyone adored. The cute bubbly little blonde was gone on the outside, but every once in a while I would see her sparkle through. But I could tell that being so sick bothered her. She didn't want to go anywhere or do anything. She didn't want anyone she didn't know to see her. She isolated herself in the back bedroom.

The COPD caused many trips to the emergency room, with her not breathing. Mostly from her sneaking out to have one puff of a cigarette. She had many visitors and she usually conned one of them into sneaking her a cigarette. I caught her once taking off her oxygen cannula, holding it at arm's length, puffing a cigarette, then putting the mask right back on. She coughed so much that she turned blue. Literally. I had to call 911.

The COPD eventually brought on congestive heart failure. It was the hardest and best time of my life. It was so sad to see her go, but at least I had the energy and felt healthy enough to be there for her. Two years earlier, it wouldn't have been the same. In fact, two years earlier, she was taking care of me.

On her deathbed, she asked me to try to quit smoking pot, with great emphasis on "smoking." She knew it helped me so she was torn. But my smoking *had* gotten out of hand. I was under so much stress; it was the only thing I could do without calling my doctor and asking for Xanax. I knew I had a problem. I just didn't know anyone else knew.

After she died, I realized I didn't want to die from smoking like her. It was the worst thing to watch happen to someone. In my nightmares I still see her gasping for breath. To see her body change the way it did, and to see her suffer, made me think. I realized I had suffered enough with M.S. and didn't want to suffer any more. And only I could change that. I had to quit smoking for *me*. When I was first diagnosed with M.S., I felt pain in places I didn't know existed. The doctors gave me pain medication, which made me feel exhausted. Wiped out. I would fall asleep and then be too tired to take care of myself, let alone my children. I hated feeling doped up all the time. So I didn't take the pain meds, and continued to feel awful.

At one of the M.S. support groups I attended, a gentleman told me he used marijuana to help manage his symptoms. He said it helped him. He explained how he could use just a little, or a lot, depending on what was happening with his symptoms. I talked to my doctor, and he told me that it did help people with M.S., but doctors were getting in trouble from the Feds for writing prescriptions for it. He wouldn't help me, for fear of the government. But another doctor I had didn't care about the politics and wrote me the prescription. I became a legal pothead.

For the first year or so, I smoked a hit or two, here and there, mostly at night to help me sleep. It helped with the few muscle spasms I still had. Then, after a while, I smoked a little more, especially when the pain was bad. I would sometimes smoke six to ten hits. Then there were times I would just smoke, to smoke. My habit began with smoking about half an ounce a month. I had a little stash carrier that held most of it, and the rest I kept in the safe. I also had a small pipe that looked like a cigarette. You seriously couldn't tell the difference. I would push the pipe into my stash and smoke my stuff anywhere I happened to be. I didn't care. It made me feel better.

I liked the fact that people thought it was cool that I got to smoke pot. I shared it with my friends. I would smoke more because I was not only smoking it for my M.S., but I was smoking it to be cool. I was smoking way more than I needed. And before long, I needed more to get the same high, or as I called it, "stabilization." Sometimes I didn't know if I was smoking to stop the pain, or if I was smoking to keep the Girl Scouts in business (I kept cases of Thin Mints and those peanut butter patties ones in my freezer).

After a couple of years, I bought a bong. As soon as the kids were asleep at night, or before they were awake in the morning, I would sit on the patio in the backyard, or in the bathroom at the window, and smoke a bong load. As the stress of my mother's illness grew, it became two bong loads. And before long, it was three. I was smoking at least three ounces of marijuana a month. But as much as I wanted to stop, I couldn't. All I could think was, "Is there enough for tomorrow?" or "Am I going to run out for my middle-of-the-night calm-me-down smoke?" The truth is, I liked how it made me feel.

I totally let the marijuana get out of hand. It was no longer just a medication to occasionally help me with my symptoms every once in a while. I was smoking it all the time. Morning noon and night. I knew it helped me with my symptoms before the transplant. But now that my symptoms were diminishing, I was still smoking just as much, if not more. I tried slowing down, but I could always find a reason to smoke. I just *loved* it. I loved being high! I finally got to the point where I realized that if I couldn't slow down, I simply had to stop.

In June of 2004, I called one of my dearest friends, Sharman, and told her how out of hand my habit had gotten. I knew she had dealt with addiction in her life and would be able to steer me in the right direction. She came right over and sat with me. She called another friend and got the name of a center where I could go. I called. They had room. I called Rob. Sharman and I played cards and just talked until Rob arrived home from work to drive me the twenty-some miles to the rehabilitation center.

"The Camp" was the name of the hellhole I stayed in while getting over my addiction (my doctor-approved legal addiction). I guess I shouldn't call it a hellhole for the sole reason it helped me (temporarily) get over my hunger for pot. But the place really was hell. I had to schlep up three flights of stairs every time I went to my room. This was not easy for someone who walked with a limp. It was also not easy because without the pot all my pain came back with a fury. It's amazing what a little marijuana can cover up.

Thanks to the "rags" you know all about Lindsay's, Whitney's, and Britney's stints in rehab. Well, now it's time to hear a little about my twenty-eight-day stint. It all began with the long silent drive to the Camp, which was in the Santa Cruz Mountains—the boondocks, Bumfuck, nowhere. Rob had noticed the pot smoking was getting out of hand and was thrilled I was doing something about it. We just did not know what to say to each other, he just held my hand. It was early evening, and Rob had just dropped me off. We had just begun to speak to each other again when they told me he had to leave; it was time to check me in. It was pitch-black outside. I cried as I filled out all the papers to be admitted. Rob was gone, and I was alone. I was sitting on a bench outside a shack, where a nurse on the inside was on the phone yelling at her daughter. She told her daughter over and over again that she had to stay home and feed her son herself, and that she was at work and couldn't help her tonight. She said this in a very loud voice, and it took over forty minutes to do so, while I sat on the bench with tears running down my face, wondering if I had made the right decision.

Just then, a young Hispanic man came over to me and asked if I was all right. Anywhere else I would have been scared to death of him. He looked like a tough guy from the East Side of San Jose. Turns out he was—from the East Side I mean. But he sat down next to me, put his arm around me, and explained that he knew exactly how I felt; he had arrived only three nights earlier. He told me that everything was going to be all right, and that God was watching and would take care of us. He then shook my hand and told me that if there was anything I needed, anything, to just ask him. His name was Marcus.

Just as the nurse decided to end her conversation with her daughter, another nurse walked up, opened the door, and walked into the shack. I heard her yell out, "Shift change." Two words I never thought I would learn to hate so much.

So after the two women went through a bunch of paperwork, caught up on how each other was, discussed the news of the day (as well as religion and politics), the original nurse finally walked out of the shack. She looked at me and said, "Oh, yeah! There's an intake out here!" She asked sweetly, "What's your name, honey?"

"Sandi," I said quietly.

"Her name is Sandi," she yelled. "Put her in 7. I haven't gone through any of her stuff." Then she walked away, not even looking back.

The second nurse walked out of the shack carrying some paperwork. She pushed her black glasses down on her nose and stared at me over them. "What ya in for?" And before I could answer, she added, "You don't look like you need detox." (Which was the nicest thing I had heard in a while.) "Come on in here; let's get you checked in."

I walked into the shack, which smelled heavily of medication. She questioned me for at least an hour, furiously writing down everything I said on her notepad. Then she took me to the laundry room, where another person went through my bags with me. He took out anything he felt was dangerous or that contained alcohol. He then assigned me my towels, bed linens, and pillow. I was then shown to my new living quarters. I sat on the bed and cried.

My roommates were great. They looked at me as though I was their little sister. They gave me hugs, showed me the ropes, and helped me adjust to my new surroundings. Those first few weeks were almost fun. We sat up talking and laughing, discussing our problems and sharing how we each should deal with them. Most of our problems were with rehab itself. The food sucked, the nurses sucked, and the people who ran it sucked. But I met some of the greatest people there.

Our complaints about rehab were real. The food was way too greasy and salty, most likely because it was the first time we'd actually tasted anything in a while. (This wasn't Betty Ford, where according to the *Enquirer*, I think it was, Wolfgang Puck stopped by to teach a pizza-making class.) The main complaint by far from nearly everyone there was about the food, but no one did anything about it. Their explanation: most people who come to rehab are malnourished and need the fat and salt. My roommates and I went so far as to watch the cooks to see why the food was so greasy. They didn't drain the meat before making spaghetti, lasagna, tacos . . .anything! It was gross.

The nurses were kind of bitchy. I didn't blame them. It couldn't be easy dealing with a bunch of addicts 24/7. But I can't tell you how many times I sat outside the shack waiting an hour, or sometimes even more, for my medication, while the nurse inside was on the phone, eating something, or just taking her dear sweet time. Then there would be a "shift change," and I had to wait for at least an hour for my medication (and several times I had to wait more than two). Somehow, they never made us wait for the food.

Here is what I learned during my stint at the Camp: I learned about addiction and control—and for that I am grateful. Now I know what to watch for in my kids, or if I start again. I also learned that having a good support group is very important. Going to the Camp's classes all day, and learning about your problems, was a wonderful way to learn to deal with your life. You can't just forget or pretend you don't have problems. The counseling helped answer why I was smoking pot: I was sick, and the pot helped. (Duh!) I also learned that depression is my trigger for abuse.

In learning about addiction, I learned that it's something passed down in families. It's genetic. Or is it? Is it in the genes, or is it a learned behavior? Either way, I didn't feel I was totally at fault. This information made me feel much better, but not as good as I felt when I was smoking pot. They also explained that overcoming addiction is something you need to work on every day, reminding yourself that you can do it. The Camp is a strong advocate of A.A., M.A., C.A., N.A. Basically anything ending with A, *anonymous*. I believe that if you need someone to lean on and make you accountable, this is the way to go. But it's not for everyone. To me, it's like church; not everyone needs to go to church to believe in God. If you have faith that you can fight your addiction, you have faith in yourself, and if your support group is strong enough, you can make it without going to meetings all the time. But either way, it's not easy. It's a daily battle. Something *you* need to keep under control. Personally I think a meeting now and then is a good reminder of what used to be.

Control is important; it is something we, as addicts, need. The more control we have, the less likely we'll be to go out and abuse again. I learned all about control at the Camp. I learned how to control my feelings and how to control the urge to use. I wanted to gain control back in my life so that I could be me again. The Camp got me started on the right road. Another reason the classes and counseling were great: they taught me how to deal with my friends and others when I returned to the *real* world. I didn't know how I was going to handle being exposed to pot again, and I knew it was going to happen.

People who were ex-users taught all the classes. Everyone who worked at the Camp was an addict, which I had mixed emotions about. Sure, they could understand everything I was going through, but they were addicts. This extends into every aspect of their lives. I know personally. We are not the most reliable people on the planet. Seriously! In fact while I was there, one of the counselors began using, and brought some back for one of the clients.

But like I said before, I made some great friends in rehab and in the aftercare, which consisted of meetings for as long as needed. These are lifelong friendships that I treasure. We may not see each other for years, but we have a bond. These are my people. We are all cut from the same cloth. We all think the same and share the same story. Addiction!

The Camp was there for me in one of my darkest hours, and for that, I will forever be grateful. It taught me that I could get clean. In fact, in June of 2007, I celebrated my three-year anniversary of being clean. I was so excited that I went out and I drank a glass of wine. I told my support group, and they told me that I was no longer clean and sober. I argued, "I never had a problem with alcohol before." But one of my friends said to me, "Hey, you never had a problem with heroin either. Why don't you do that?" I got the message. But heroin will never be a problem for me—remember, I hate needles. One thing I have realized, though, is that a glass of wine once a month won't kill me, and if I'm no longer considered sober, that is okay with me. Give me the pot.

I support the medical use of marijuana. I think it's important for people to be able to choose for themselves what works for them. I know for a fact, it worked for me. I just wish someone would put THC in an inhaler. That would be brilliant!

Chapter 8
Now What?

Sure, my stem cell transplant worked. It worked a little too well I might add. Because all of a sudden, my body began rejecting all foreign objects. First it was my husband, then a piece of pencil lead from my arm (I remember—sixth grade—Mike Smith). Then a rock came out of my knee. I was shocked! I thought there would've been a lot more with the amount of time I spent on my knees in high school. Hey! Get your mind out of the gutter. I was praying. Yeah, praying my father wouldn't find out about all the guys I was doing.

Since my stem cell transplant, I can honestly say my body has changed in ways I never thought imaginable. Menopause being the first of many side effects from chemo and radiation. It would be hard for anybody to conceive all the different things that were happening to my body, unless you were standing here and looking at things from my view. Everything has gotten so much better, although in some ways, things have become quite strange. Sure, my M.S. is at bay, but some things that have come up have scared the hell out of me.

After the transplant, I felt different right away. Weird things began happening to me. I knew I was getting better because my body began spitting out foreign objects—and I mean actual things from under my skin. You might wonder, "What kind of foreign objects might you have in your body, Sandi?" First, there was a piece of pencil lead in my right arm. Several weeks later, my body spat out a piece of lava rock, then a rock from my eye, and last but not least, my breast implants.

So, the lead. I had always had this dark spot on my right arm. I never even thought about it until June 1st, when my arm began to swell. Then it began to ache. Red streaks began shooting up my arm and into my chest. When I squeezed my arm, it turned white. It was so gross. It was like a huge pimple. I scratched at the surface. Then I poked it with a needle, and out came a slimy green puss-covered bump. *Very* gross! But in the middle of the green was something black. Turns out it was a pencil lead.

I remember being stabbed (by accident) in the sixth grade by Mike Smith. I remembered when I was in sixth grade; my mother bought me the cutest loose-knit white sweater. It was way cool! It was my first day wearing it to school. Mike Smith had just sharpened his pencil at the pencil sharpener. I sat just five steps away from the sharpener. He was there for what seemed like an hour getting that super-fine tip. Then Mr. Marshall yelled for him to hurry back to his seat. As he went by my seat, he caught his super-fine sharpened pencil in my brand-new sweater. It punched right through and into my arm. I don't think he even noticed when it happened, at least not until he sat down to write and realized the super-fine tip was somehow missing.

Hey Mike, I found it!

And the rock. In the middle of July, my left knee began to swell. It was the same thing. My knee was twice its normal size. Rob thought I must have fallen and hurt it. But I didn't remember falling. Now I knew the drill. I could see the red streaks up and down my leg all leading to a small white area. Again, I scratched the surface, and again, a small item came out from under the skin, surrounded by a green film and puss. This turned out to be a tiny piece of lava rock, *red lava rock*, just like the one in front of my neighbor's house in Almaden. One that I never could quite jump all the way over when I was ten. You can still see the original scar from when I hit the rock. Yeah, I remember that rock.

At the end of July, my left eye began to swell. Same drill. Only this one hurt a lot more than the other two. I literally had a bubble over my left eye. I poked around and finally it popped out. Out came something encapsulated in green. It looked like a small brown piece of dirt.

Then I remembered that when I was three years old, I was hit in the eye by a rock. A boy in our neighborhood with only two fingers on his right hand, whom we so lovingly called "Teddy Two Fingers" threw it at me. Now you know why he was so angry and throwing rocks—because we called him "Teddy Two Fingers"! For some reason, he threw a rock at me, and it cut my eye open right above the brow. I had several stitches, but there must have been just a little piece of dirt left in there to fester all these years.

In January of 2001, my right breast began to ache. It swelled until it was twice the size of the left one. There were red streaks going down my arm, and I was thinking that *this* wasn't going to be quite so easy. A little scratch won't help here. I ended up in the emergency room that evening, having my right breast implant removed. Yes! Get rid of them! I had thought they were going to make me happy. I realized a little too late that wasn't the case. But boy, were they fun while they lasted!

The doctor called my insurance company and asked if they should remove both implants since it seemed obvious my body would reject the other one too. The insurance company said, "No. Wait until it is necessary." Hello? *I* think it is necessary! I personally did not want to walk around like Quasi Mama until the next one decided to blow! I begged the insurance company. They still said no. So the doctors did what the insurance company said and kept the left one in. I still can't believe I walked around afterwards with one huge breast and one not-so-huge breast.

But it only took a month, almost to the day, and I was back in the emergency room. Sorry, Mr. Insurance Man, now it's going to cost you double.

I was dealing with insurance and death. First, it was my mother then a month to the day after my mother died, my aunt followed. What was even more depressing…my grandmother passed away one year later. I couldn't imagine watching my children go before me.

During this time, I was serving on the board of the National M.S. Society. I was hoping I could give them some information about what I had been through, and what my stem cell transplant did for me. I wanted to give the information to those that wanted it; for those looking for something more extreme, I knew it worked. The woman running our local chapter knew it worked. She finally asked me to write an article about stem cell research and about my transplant. She told me that they were going to print it in their paper because she had seen the change in me and knew it worked. Six months later, I gave up asking when the article was going to be published. But just like everything else there, I was told it was held up by red tape; it was with the lawyers.

Everyone there saw how much I had improved. I was traveling again. Rob's new boss and his wife took us with them to the Grammys several years in a row. I could fly on a plane without using every barf bag in my row. We traveled a lot with my husband's new boss Mike Homer from Kontiki, his wife Kristina, their family Scott and Shari, and M.C. Hammer (or, as he goes by now, Hammer) and his amazing wife Stephanie. Kontiki was a start-up company that did streamline videos. Hammer wanted to utilize Kontiki's processes for his music, so we spent a lot of time together. During this time I was feeling better than I had in years. And it was so nice to be around families that are into *their* family. Thanks to the Homers and Hammers, I have some of the best memories I could ever hope for. I was getting better by the day.

But back at the M.S. Society…The way I saw it, if the article didn't appeal to the masses, it wasn't supported by the Society, especially if it was about a new treatment not supported by the drug companies. They weren't in the business of telling you what could be; they just wanted to give you the facts of what you already knew. They didn't want to anger their main sponsors, the companies who make M.S. drugs. I think the drug companies would stop supporting them. And I think the drug companies have the final say on *everything*.

Here is my personal example: I had been doing stand-up comedy for about two years at local clubs, joking about my life. I had offered my services to help with a fundraiser for our local chapter. I was the chairperson in charge. I was also going to perform at the fundraiser. It was going to be a comedy fundraiser. We had talked about getting other local comedians in the area to help out, but the local chapter decided to get Teri Garr. I was thrilled. She'd starred in *Young Frankenstein* and *Tootsie*. She also has M.S. We were going to do a show at a local downtown hotel. It was going to be a luncheon. We called it "Lunch and Laughter with Teri Garr," and in small type, "and Sandi Selvi."

I was going to open for Teri Garr! I can't tell you how excited I was. They gave me Teri's manager's phone numbers and email address. I immediately wrote her manager and told her how excited I was. I also told her that I had been through a stem cell transplant and would love to talk to Teri about it. Her manager called me and told me that they were looking forward to the show, and she would be in touch with me beforehand. I was so excited that I purchased three tables to seat all my family and friends. Three tables, at $5,000 apiece (and that didn't even include the chairs).

Three days before the show, the M.S. Society called me and told me that Teri Garr's "people" wanted to know exactly, word for word, what I was going to say. They wanted it written down, in script form, and sent to them. They would read it over and let me know the day of the show if they would allow me to even go on. They didn't like the fact that my whole routine centered on and around my stem cell transplant. They didn't think that what I had to say would fit in with what Teri had to say. They also made it clear that they didn't think comedy and M.S. mixed well together. Then why were we calling the thing "Lunch and LAUGHTER with Teri Garr"?

What I was not told was that Teri's "people" were the drug company that sponsored her. I don't even know if Teri knew what they did to me. It was *my* fundraiser and *I* was the chairperson. I even donated $15,000 to it. I was bumped out because the drug company didn't like what I had to say. They did not want stem cell research talked about while Teri was using their drug. The drug company sponsored more things for the M.S. Society than I did. So I was out.

Right after the Terri Garr incident, I ended up in rehab. Right after rehab I began having stomach pains. It was my gallbladder. The pot was no longer masking the pain. When they took it out, they found it riddled with vasculitis, a new autoimmune disorder. Disease #352! Okay, it wasn't really disease #352, it was disease #353, or at least it seemed like it. But if I had still been high from smoking pot, I don't know if I would have ever noticed that sort of pain. Come to find out, it could have killed me. Vasculitis is the thickening of the veins, and it can be deadly. So far, thank goodness, that's the only place they've found it. And then they took it out.

Not having a gallbladder has been a strange experience. I used to love ice cream, creamed sauces, coffee with milk, and cheese. Without a gallbladder, all these things I used to love now give me stomach pains. If I continue to eat them in the quantities I used to enjoy, I get sick. By cutting down on all these fatty foods I loved so much, I have also cut down on my weight too! Bonus!

It took a while to realize it, but I had also developed a thyroid problem from the radiation treatment I received during my transplant. At first, I had hypothyroidism, or Hashimoto's. Disease #354! My thyroid was working very slowly. Okay, let's be honest, it was basically not working at all. I was tired all the time. I had gained a lot of weight and wasn't feeling like myself. I was almost a hundred and fifty pounds, which I had not been since I was pregnant. So they put me on Synthroid.

The medication helped a little, but I still felt horrible.

Sometimes I was jittery, and sometimes I was sluggish. Then my stem cells kicked in, and my thyroid began working on its own again (but only while I was on medication). I guess it just needed a *little* stimulation, because it began working a little too well—so well that I became hyperthyroid. I was then diagnosed with Graves' disease (#355!). My thyroid was working way too much, especially because I was still on the medication for hypothyroidism. I was anxious all the time, couldn't sleep, shook like I'd drunk way too much coffee, and I was losing weight *fast*. I was down to a hundred and twelve pounds at one point.

My doctor changed my medication again. My thyroid went back to not working. I gained thirty-five pounds right away. They changed my medication again and the Graves' came back. My doctor and I worked on it for four years and couldn't get it right. My body began to produce an antibody, which began attaching to the tissue behind my eyes. The doctor says the tissue behind the eyes very closely resembles the thyroid tissue, and the antibodies can't tell the difference. So the antibodies attacked the tissue behind the eyes, which caused the tissue to swell. I began to look like the freaky love child of Betty Davis and Marty Feldman.

My eyes stuck out so far that when I wore my glasses, my eyes actually touched the lenses. The pressure pushing my eyes out was stretching the optic nerve. I was going blind. I had tunnel vision and sometimes couldn't see anything. I became depressed and angry, mostly because I was scared; I went in search of pot. I was back on a medical roller-coaster. I would sit at home and cry, and I couldn't explain why I was crying. This damn thing turned me into a depressed Country Western singer. "Just two big bulging eyes, crying in the rain." No one knew what to do with me. Rob would tell me to stop crying, but I didn't know how. So I began renting sad movies, any tearjerker I could find. This way, I knew what I was crying about. It let me have some form of control. I smoked a little pot. It at least stopped the pain, and I slept like a baby.

I finally ended up at UCSF to have my thyroid checked. At first, the doctors there were going to do radiation and try to kill my thyroid. Since medication hadn't been able to stabilize it in four years, they thought it was time to do something "a little more drastic." I think killing it is pretty drastic. Then I talked to the doctors at the Scripps Center in San Diego, where I'd had my transplant, which would require about the three months of steroids that I would have to be on to protect my eyes from getting any worse. They all decided that it would be too dangerous to my immune system. It could possibly bring my multiple sclerosis back into play. Ha! Not going to happen.

Okay. What else could we do?

Surgery.

SURGERY?

What? The past eighteen surgeries haven't been enough? Seriously, eighteen surgeries. I gave a list of what I thought were all seventeen of them to the doctor. I had them all organized by date, surgery type, and location of surgery. A computer-generated list. All seventeen. My doctor's assistant exclaimed, "Wow! Seventeen surgeries. I've only had one my entire life." She waited a second and then went on, "I had my tonsils out when I was a kid."

I grabbed the paper away from the doctor and said, "Sorry. Tonsils removed, 1963, San Jose, California. I didn't know that was considered a real surgery." That made it a whopping eighteen. The thyroid surgery would make it my nineteenth surgery. The doc said it would only be a small incision in my neck.

The surgery went well. It was supposed to take an hour. It took almost four. Because I use my voice for my work, they wanted to be extra careful around my vocal cords. So the incision ended up being much bigger than planned. The thyroid had grown right against the vocal cords, and it was difficult to remove.

My throat hurt constantly for two weeks following that surgery. My voice sounded like Stewart on MAD TV for almost two months, all high-pitched and whispery. Then, all of a sudden, it began to get low and gravelly. Some say sexy; I say I sounded like I had smoked five or six packs of cigarettes with a cold. It took almost four months for my voice to get back to normal, and eight months longer than that to get the medication right. So, as soon as the doctor had the medication for my thyroid just right (and sometimes I wonder about that!), I got to look forward to surgery number twenty. And "look" is just a figure of speech because I couldn't see anything. My eyes were so bugged out of my head that everything in front of me was blurred, and everything to the sides of me was double (which was totally opposite from my M.S. days) and everything was slowly going black.

I knew something was wrong when my vision started going dark all the time. The bulging was making my eyes stick out so far that it was pulling on my optic nerve. I was going to go blind if I didn't do something. The thought of eye surgery bothered me a little. Screw that, it bothered me a lot! I am a visual person. I need my eyes. The doctor was going to have to cut through *something*, take out, and *I don't know* la, la, la, la. Something about waking me up during surgery to adjust the muscle by pulling in a suture. But mostly all I heard in my head was la, la, la, la. I didn't want to know. I was so scared. I asked if I was going to be asleep through the entire process. Then I asked if the surgeon knew what she was doing. Then I asked what she thought my chances of survival were. Her answers: Yes, and 99 percent. Good. After that I didn't want to hear any more about what they were going to do. As long as I was going to be asleep, I was good to go. Just do it!

The surgery lasted eight hours. The Graves' disease had made the material behind my eyes so built up that it had cut off my sinuses. I also had a deviated septum and an infection that had been there for over a year (an infection that eight antibiotics and steroids hadn't been able to kill). The infection had begun to go into my right ear. It was both painful and strange. There was so much fluid, I had begun to lose hearing in that ear. My balance was way off. And let's not forget my eyes. I *had* to have the surgery.

And it went well, as far as my sinuses and ear were concerned. My eyes were another story. This is what the surgeon tried to explain to me earlier. I should have listened.

Do you know what she did to me? She cut two slits by my eyes. They weren't small little slits; they had to be big enough to be able to get to the bone (the bone on the outside of my eye socket, right next to my temple). They needed to get that bone out of the way. They just broke it! Took the bone out, so they could take my eyes out of my head. OH YEAH, they took my eyes out of my head! Took all the material behind my eyes out and then put my eyes back in. *Gross!*

I went home looking like a prizefighter after twelve hard rounds. All around my eyes, it was red and swollen, and in some areas it was black and blue. My eyes were so swollen, the eyelids were transparent and turned inside out. The whites of my eyes were now bright red; the white had been replaced with blood. I was unrecognizable. I took pictures. I look back now and remember: it was scary!

My eyes didn't go back where they were supposed to go. I don't remember being woken up during surgery to have my eyes adjusted. I do remember *that* part of the conversation prior to the surgery. It never happened.

So, during my convalescence, I remember at one point thinking something went really wrong. Then I noticed my right eye was facing a little straighter forward than my left eye. My left eye was looking directly at my nose, and the right eye wasn't exactly "right" either. It was hard to notice because I couldn't see very well. My eyes weren't able to focus on anything, having just been taken out of my head and all. Sure, I still had 20/20 vision in each eye, but they just weren't able to focus on the same thing at the same time. I thought the swelling might have something to do with it, but when the doctors came in to visit me, they explained what had happened.

My eyes had crossed. The right eye settled back in the eye socket correctly, while the left eye did not. CROSSED EYES? What next? Oh yeah, I forgot. I have to quit asking that question because every time I do, I get an answer. They wanted to wait until all the swelling from this surgery had gone down, to do the next surgery. The doctor knew there would be another surgery already? Shit. They put me on short bursts of prednisone to help the swelling go down more quickly. The surgery was scheduled for three weeks later, two days before my oldest son's high school graduation. We were cutting it close. *Cutting*. Surgery. Get it? Oh yes, I used that on stage. I had to laugh about it, otherwise I would cry. I was sick of crying. It hurt to cry.

There I was at UCSF, in the surgery center, facing surgery number twenty- two. Well, my right eye was facing it; my left eye was watching a young intern bend over. My eyes weren't right, but they were better. I was lying on the gurney; the I.V. had just been put in. My heart felt like it was beating out of my chest, and my blood pressure had skyrocketed to 104 over 64 (normal for me is 90/60). The anesthesiologist was standing over me with what he called the "happy juice," which was going to make me comfortable before I went into the surgery room.

Just then, the doctor arrived. She took one look at me and said, "Stop everything!" She did a few tests and went on to tell me that I looked great, and she didn't think surgery would be neces- sary. But I still saw double! The tests showed that my eyes were twice as good as they were three weeks earlier. She rated my eyes a ten, and said they only had to be a six for the brain to kick in and fix the rest. I thought that meant they were ten degrees off and had to get to six degrees. Maybe this is where the saying "six degrees of separation" originally comes from. I was quickly on my way to having normal eyesight without surgery. Yeah!

She wanted me to see her two weeks later, which would give her a better idea of whether I would ever need eye surgery again or not. The best explanation she could give me now for not doing the surgery was: if I did it, a month or so later, I might have to go back and correct it the other way. Good enough for me, I thought, but can I still have the "happy juice"? Surgery or not, it had been a rough day. And when I did in fact ask for the "happy juice," they all laughed like I was joking and then set me free.

I underwent all that surgery because of my thyroid. Thyroids are strange. So much depends on a balanced thyroid. I can honestly say having a hyper thyroid is much more uncomfortable than having a hypo thyroid. I know! It was a four-year roller-coaster ride I wouldn't wish on anyone. Okay, maybe one person, and she knows who she is.

I really wasn't looking forward to another surgery, or two, so soon. So I was happy they didn't have to do the second surgery. The left eye was painful when I tried to look left. But I could deal with that, especially because I had found pot in my son's room. What was he going to do, tell my husband? "Dad, Mom stole my pot."

If you have lost track, and want to be in the know, this is a list of the surgeries I've had so far. Beginning now with #1: Tonsils removed.

#	Date	Surgery
1.	March 1963	Tonsils removed
2.	Dec. 1979	Appendix removed
3.	June 1990	Breast implants, silicon
4.	Jan. 1991	Breast implants, saline
5.	March 1991	Cyst ovary & tubes tied
6.	Dec. 1991	Back L4, L5 discectomy
7.	Dec. 1992	Back L4, L5 framinotomy/discectomy
8.	Feb. 1994	Right torn rotator cuff in shoulder
9.	July 1995	Sinus polyps removed
10.	April 1996	Right elbow torn tendon

11. June 1996	Broken nose fixed
12. March 16, 2000	Mediport in chest
13. March 17, 2000	Punctured lung re-inflated
14. March 31, 2000	Stem cell transplant
15. Jan. 2001	R breast implant removed
16. Feb. 2001	L breast implant removed
17. Nov. 2003	Cyst removed from face
18. Feb. 2005	Gallbladder removed
19. Nov. 2005	Thyroid removed
20. May 11, 2006	Eye decompression, Graves'
21. May 11, 2006	Sinus & deviated septum

Twenty-one surgeries, at least that was what I thought until my "Girl Friday" (Katelyn) mentioned she was shocked that with all I had had done surgically, wisdom teeth extraction was not on my list. She was facing that herself the following week. Which reminded me…

| 22. August 1978 | Wisdom Teeth Extraction |

So on the calendar, Wisdom Teeth Extraction is actually surgery # 2. For those still counting. I will fix the order later.

Plus, I thought the surgeries would end there. But I was seeing double, even with glasses. My left eye was fixed on my nose, and nothing could catch its attention. Believe me, Rob tried. Then the pain began. I was told to wear an eyepatch. I bought a patch. It was an ugly black patch from the pharmacy. Rob got on the Internet and bought me some cool ones at a place called www.eyepatchheaven.com. One had dice, one had flames, one had butterflies. Rob is the sweetest man on the planet.

But eventually, I had to have the eye fixed. It only kept getting worse, and I was getting sick of the double vision. It had gotten to the point where I would throw up when I opened both eyes at the same time.

23. July 2006   Fix lazy eye

The doctor had told me they were going to wake me up during surgery to adjust the muscle. But when I woke up, I realized they hadn't. The doctor told me she thought she calculated it correctly once she saw what she was dealing with. She moved the eye the correct number of degrees. There was no need to wake me. At the time I thought, Maybe there *is* a God. And after my surgery, my left eye seemed to be better. I hate that word "seemed," but it really seemed better. I could now look left. And new glasses helped. With my prism glasses, there was no more double vision. These glasses had a prism set in to the lens that made my eye see ten degrees off, lining up my eyes perfectly. People commented on how cute they were. Best of all, I could see! But as time went by, my left eye began giving me problems again. Even the glasses weren't helping. I could no longer look left or up. And when I tried, I would get vertigo. Where were those patches?

My eye had to be fixed again. The muscles didn't attach correctly. My left eye was looking at my nose.

24. April 2007   Fix lazy eye, again

I remember waking up during *that* surgery. They sat me upright, a nurse on each side of the doctor in front of me. They had me look at something (I can't remember what), to see if it was double. YES, it was. They pulled a string attached to the muscle in my eye, which in my head sounded like a rope being dragged against a ship hull. All while I sat there. AWAKE! I could feel it every time they pulled. And they pulled just a little bit at a time, for what seemed like an hour. I was supposed to tell them when I thought things looked straight. I was drugged and a little creeped out. I had a date like that once. I wonder if I was the best judge of what was straight anyways. As Rob would say, "Isn't there anyone here a little more qualified?"

When we were all satisfied with the straightness, the doctor came at me with a pair of scissors to cut the rope hanging out of my eye. What was left in my eye was now my suture. I was glad they were laying me back down. I would have looked stupid when I passed out, which I was about to do. So, using a whole roll of white paper tape, they fastened a steel eyepatch to my face and sent me on my way.

Things went great for almost a year. Then I noticed a change in my left eye again. It was getting harder to look left and up again. A few weeks later, it began to get hard to look down. Then my eye just froze in one place. I couldn't look left, up, down, or right. If I tried, I would throw up. We had to do something quick. I know, the old "wake me up, rope in the eye" routine. Get it over with!

25. July 2008   Fix lazy eye, again

This surgery didn't go as well as we had expected. They didn't wake me up during surgery this time like they said they would. Something had gone very wrong. When my eye was healing from the last surgery, the scar tissue caused the muscles to attach completely around the eye. It wasn't supposed to do that. Doctors had to cut away most of the muscle to put my eye back in place. The muscles were so short now that my left eye couldn't work in tandem with my right eye.

This surgery made my double vision even worse than it had been in the past. Before, I could wear glasses to fix the vertical degree of separation. Now, my left eye was seeing everything at a slant, horizontally, while my right eye saw everything straight. When I closed my right eye, everything appeared to be going downhill. When I closed my left eye, everything was right again. Not only was the vision from the left eye tipped, but there was also still a separation between my eyes, vertically. Vertical and horizontal differences together, a combination glasses cannot fix. I know—we've tried.

I could only find one of the old eyepatches Rob had bought me from the last surgery. The flames. I discovered that the kids had used the other ones for Halloween costumes: one was a pirate; the other was a rabbi (he used it as a yarmulke). They also used them as slingshots, and I swear I saw my son's girlfriend swimming with a pair of them as her bathing suit top. My husband got back on the website looking for more eyepatches. He helped me pick out different shapes, sizes, and colors. Yippee! New accessories!

One of the downfalls of this situation was that getting to comedy might be difficult. I can't drive at night. And the patch makes it hard to see things. It doesn't matter which side I wear it on, I still have 20/20 vision in each eye. Collectively they are a mess. You can tell. Just look at the left side of my garage. Yes, I hit it. And don't forget about the falling. I kept tripping over things and falling down. Landing on my butt. Sometimes I can't see things with the patch on, it kind of blocks my vision. I call it my eyepatch blind spot. Small running children may be cute to some. They're a *hazard* to me. And don't get me started about the animals being walked down the street on a leash. I can't see them or their leashes. And on those streets, there is a curb. *That* was my second fall. It's not safe out there. Monk is right; it's a jungle out there!

My doctor suggested I see a therapist, to see if we could get the eyes to work together again. I thought it worked for my husband and me. Why not? So I began eye therapy. Yeah, I had no idea eye therapy existed either. But it does, and it works. When I started therapy, I had to be within a foot of your face to see you. Anything beyond that was double, and if I tried to look closer I would get nauseous; sometimes I would just throw up. I couldn't use my computer. Even with an eyepatch I would get sick to my stomach. Between that and the pain from behind my eyes, there was no way I could have finished this book. But thanks to Dr. Kageyama and Dr. Shao, my therapists, I can see up to eighteen feet before things go double. And if I keep going it may get even better.

I no longer need my patch around the house. But as soon as I go out the door on to unfamiliar territory, I have to put it on. If people are going to stare, I would rather it be at the eyepatch than me on the ground. It cuts the chance of me falling by almost half.

It was hard for me to look down. The next fall happened for other reasons. (The third time was definitely not a charm.) I was at the spa and needed to wear my eyepatch. I didn't see the ledge on the side of the walkway. It was in my eyepatch blind spot. My new favorite saying when anything goes wrong now is "I can't see!" And I really didn't see the ledge so I fell. My friend stopped me from falling all the way down. She grabbed my arm, and I felt a twinge in my shoulder when I stopped. The same shoulder I had been avoiding seeing the doctor about for years. Pop!

It hurt so much that I couldn't raise my arm, so it was a pain in the ass. Not literally. But enough for me to give in, and call a doctor. I had an MRI. Met with the doctor. Turns out, I have a calcium deposit in my shoulder that's causing inflammation, so Dr. Delaney gave me a cortisone shot. Just like that. He pointed to where he was going to do it and then he just did it! Like that. I passed out. I hate it when that happens. The second I saw the needle in my shoulder, I remember looking at Rob and saying, "You'd better get over here, I think I'm going to . . ." and that was all I got out before he saw my eyes roll back in my head. Which he caught very nicely against his chest. The next thing I remember was Rob saying, "Don't worry, I have you." Like I said, he is my rock!

The cortisone worked for a few weeks, after that it lacked it's ability to stop me from throttling someone, just from me trying to comb my own hair. The pain was that intense.

26. October 2, 2009   Left Shoulder, Calcium deposit
                        removed rotator repair

Surgery number twenty-six went better than expected. A small calcium deposit was scraped off and a stitch was put in my rotator cuff, it was a small tear. But as simple as the procedure was, it was my 26th surgery. I had read an article that said statistically speaking one out of every twenty-six surgeries ended in a cataclysmic event, i.e. death being the one that caught my eye. I was sure that this was going to be the one, until my friend Judy (yes! the same Judy from elementary school/Barbies/First communion), reminded me about the whole lung puncture thing, and said, "Some people would put that in the category of cataclysmic." She had a point! But I have to admit I was still a little nervous going in.

My eyes are getting better but I still have double vision at a distance, so I still wear the patch when I am away from home. Still having problems looking down, the eyes just don't want to work together. So, I began doing puzzles with my friend Judy, and Judy's friend from work, now my friend, Victoria. It seems to be helping. We call it puzzle therapy.

Chapter 9
Won't Do Stand-Up in a Wheelchair

I've been traveling a lot for my comedy gigs. After 9-11, and all the crap since then, I was nervous about traveling, but my husband told me not to worry. He said he'd be following me with his heart. But I think he is actually having me followed. All the way to the airport there was a line of cars, and in the security line, there were tons of people behind me. When I went to the airport map to find my gate, there was a red dot with the words 'You Are Here' right under it. How did he know?

After my stem cell transplant, while I was recuperating from the chemotherapy and radiation, all I did was listen to comedy tapes. I'm still convinced the first one, by Brian Regan, saved my life. When friends called to say they wanted to stop by, they'd ask if I needed anything. I would say, "No flowers. Doctors' rules. But could you pick me up a comedy tape?" Comedy honestly got me through the hardest times. Laughter made me feel good. Because I wasn't able to be around others, I would sit there with my headphones on giggling to myself. Sometimes I would even laugh out loud.

When I was able to be around people and do the things I wanted to do again, I decided that I would pursue comedy, I wanted to become a stand-up comedian. If I was going to live—and that was indeed in question at times—I wanted to feel good all the time. And comedy made me feel good all the time. I wanted it in my life.

I stopped renting sad movies. I was sick and tired of crying all the time. I was sick and tired of being sick and tired. I rented every funny movie I could find, and I listened to comedy night and day, day and night. After a while I thought, "I am so much funnier than all these guys." I had been making people laugh since I was a kid, and I loved to tell stories. I also loved to get up in front of people and talk. Hell, I just loved to talk. And if tragedy is comedy, I was born to be a comedian.

I remember in junior high, I was running for school secretary, and I had to give a speech. I knew I had no way of winning the race because I was running against one of the most popular girls in school. I had already signed up, however, and was too embarrassed to just drop out, so I gave it a whirl. I enlisted my next-door neighbor, Nanci, the funniest person I knew, to co-write the speech with me. If I was going out, I was going out laughing. So my speech began like this: "Hi, I'm Sandi. I am running for secretary. I am so quick, some people refer to me as Secretariat." I gave myself the appropriate few-second pause to hear all the laughter. Sure, all the teachers, and a few of the proud parents who came to hear their children speak, chuckled, but all the kids in the room just sat there kicking their chairs, with their mouths closed and blank looks on their faces. I could barely go on, but I did, and NO, I did not win. Little did I know I was setting myself up for the big stage!

In April of 2001, I decided to look for a place where I could study comedy. I got on the Internet and found a few places that taught comedy classes, but the San Francisco Comedy College stuck out in particular, mostly because they had a location just a few blocks from my house. They also asked the same two questions I was asking myself: Was I as funny as I thought? Could I be funnier?

It didn't take me long to realize that YES! I am funny! I have a rich life filled with tragedy to draw real comedy from. Comedy and tragedy walk the same line. This is what I have learned makes me laugh, and what most drives my comedy. It has to be real, and I am as real as they come.

I am not a fan of hack comedy. I hate it when a comedian gets on stage and does the equivalent of poop jokes, or what I refer to as Popsicle shtick comedy (something they read off a Popsicle stick). They tell one joke after another that doesn't tie the comedian to anything. These are the shows people walk out of and can't remember any real thing about the comedian. You might be able to remember one or two of their jokes, but not their name or who they were.

If comedy doesn't come from the heart, and is not a real part of you, you can't get attached to it, and people will not believe it's the real you. Sure, you can be gimmicky or tell one joke after another with no truth behind it, but people eventually will see through that and want to know who you are. People like a story. Something they can connect with.

One of the gals from the comic troupe 3 Blonde Moms told a group of us once, "Know who you really are comically. While you're listening to comedy, every time you laugh out loud, write down what the joke was about. After watching and listening to several hours of comedy, you should have a pretty good idea of what makes you laugh."

I learned that the kind of comedy you enjoy is the kind of comedy you should be doing. Don't waste your time with comedy that will just make you feel okay and wanting more. There is not enough time in the day to waste on bad comedy.

The San Francisco Comedy College (SFCC), and its founder Kurtis Matthews, taught me a lot. I will never forget my first day of school. We met at the Los Gatos History Club in Los Gatos. There were six people in the beginners' class with me. Five of them have remained my close friends to this day. Which is great because comedy is a funny business (and not always in a good way). People come and go faster than the counter girl at Nordstrom's.

At first, the class would learn the fundamentals of joke writing. Find a premise. Ask yourself, "What is the logical conclusion to the premise?" Now, go in the opposite direction. You have a joke. Sounds simple, but it's not. Now, get a bunch of those "jokes" and link them together through segues. It really isn't as easy as it sounds. Then it would help if you have a few callbacks, which are links from one joke to another by either using the same punch line for unrelated jokes, or the same premise. Not an easy thing to do at all.

We sat around listening to each other do comedy. Then Kurtis, the guy who ran the school, told us what he liked and what he didn't like. Some of the class members also would put in their two cents. It was fun.

After a few months, I moved on to the advanced class. I was so excited. We joined the other people who had actually been on stage and doing comedy for months. Some of them had even been doing it for years. Our class grew to a whopping thirteen. (This didn't last long. A lot of people start out in this business, but not a lot of people stay. There are two reasons for this: number one, it's hard, and number two, there's no money in it.) The older people seemed so seasoned. It was so much fun to do our bits and get feedback from the ones who'd been in the business for what seemed like such a long time. Turns out, a couple of years is kind of like dipping your toe in the ocean. A good start.

After my second month of taking classes, I went on stage for the first time. I performed at Waves Steakhouse. It was an experience that changed my life. The house was packed, not all of them to see comedy, most were just eating their dinners. I was so nervous. I had bought a dress to perform in and had to go out and change because I wet my pants. My husband was there alone, sitting next to the wife of one of the other guys from class. I talked about my sons being a pain in the ass, and all about me confusing MS and S&M. When I heard the roar of laughter, I felt more alive than I ever had. As soon as I was finished, I wanted to do it again and again.

I continued going to class. Once a week, we worked really

hard on our bits. We talked about all the open mics in the area, and where we could try out our new comedy. On the nights we weren't in class, we were at comedy clubs, nightclubs, pizza joints, and in people's backyards—anywhere and everywhere we could do comedy. Once a month, we had a graduation night. It was at a venue where we could all go and perform our latest stuff. I did this for years, performing for free anywhere I could.

Then I began to wonder, where were the big bucks?

Since no one knew me yet, I had to perform for free. It was the only way to get on stage. Most of the time, I had to pay for my parking and food, so it was costing me. But I loved every minute of it and didn't care. I was motivated and I just wanted to make people laugh. All of them. All of the time. I performed at coffeehouses, restaurants, bars, and charity events. I did not want to see one blank face starring back at me, and definitely no one bored enough to be kicking their chair. It was working. I made them laugh. Me!

Since I've been performing, I've met some of the most awesome people I never otherwise would have encountered. Some of these people I will stay friends with until the day I die. Sure, they aren't as funny as I am, but I still like them.

After a few years with the Comedy College, I started going on field trips to New York (twice), Arizona (twice), and Los Angeles (three times). I performed in showcases at Rooster T. Feathers in Sunnyvale, and the IMPROVs in San Jose, Tempe, and Hollywood. While in New York, I performed at Stand Up New York, Caroline's, and the Cellar. Then I was asked by Maria Bamford herself to do a guest set at the Punch Line in San Francisco. Maria was and still is one of the funniest women in comedy. She is insane. And I respected that insanity the way I respect Robin Williams. That, to me, was the coolest thing that had ever happened and the highest form of compliment. I had a great show. Since then she has asked me to open for her every time she's in town. It feels good!

I love comedy. I love being on stage and hearing laughter. I also love laughing. People always ask who I like and who inspired me. Here are just a few: Mitch Hedberg,, Richard Prior, Richard Belzer, Chris Rock, Maria Bamford, Alonzo Bodden, Ray Romano, Will Durst, Ellen DeGeneres, Kevin James, and Brian Regan. Since I've been doing comedy, my list has grown even more to include a few local talents. I love Sammy Obeid, Sharman Summers, Lynn Ruth Miller, Sandy Stec, Beth Schumann, Jeff Applebaum, Maggie Newcomb, Bob Brindley, Mike Holly, Sal Calani, Reggie Steele, Johnny Steele, John DeKoven, Mari Esther Kaplan, Tim Babs, Tammy Shea, Ricky Stimbra, Sammy Saifir, Joe Gleckler, Dan Edwards, Robert Peterson, Gary Penovich, and my most favorite comedian of all, Joe Klocek. To me, Joe is what funny is all about. Just like Richard and Mitch before him, when I think of Joe Klocek, I think Quick-wit. Some of these people are seriously funny. I have performed with all of them, some I know from the Comedy College (SFCC), and I have seen a lot of comedians. I have struggled with a few to get jobs, rides, write. These are my friends and you will inevitably see their names on a comedy club marquee someday (in small letters) just under mine.

I love almost everything about this business except maybe for the favoritism shown to male comics versus female comics. Everybody talks about it; nobody does anything to change it. Other than the fact that most clubs are run by men, I have no idea why they don't like women. Most likely it's because most of us won't will sleep with them, well then again, some do, and you know who you are. The rest of us have to be that much more funny.

Oh! And I hate it when people don't laugh. This has happened on occasion. Sure, they might not laugh at all my jokes, but I've always been able to get the audience to laugh at least a little, if not all the way through my performance. But one day— okay, it was in May 2005—I was invited to do a benefit show in a restaurant in the mountains. I won't say where. What the promoter didn't tell us before lining up the gig was that the audience consisted primarily of lesbians. Okay, that was an understatement. There were one hundred and eight people in the restaurant that day, and the only people who weren't gay were the five performers. Yes, even the restaurant owners were lesbians. I have nothing against lesbians, just the ones at the show who didn't laugh. It seemed like they all hated us. Not one of them laughed through all five performers. I will never forget one woman walking up to the performer right in front of me and saying, "Aren't any of you funny?" I was up next and just wanted to crawl into a hole. They wanted lesbian comedy. They did not want to hear about my sons, dumb and dumber.

In spite of what the lesbians thought, I knew I had to take my comedy to the next level. I began taking comedy classes from anyone and everyone. While continuing classes at SFCC, I took classes from Steven Rosenfield at the American Comedy Institute in New York, and from Heather at Rooster T. Feathers in Sunnyvale, CA.

I felt that if I learned everything they all knew, I could pick and choose what worked for me. It worked. It got me more shows and got me to expand my comedy a little. But I still wasn't confident enough on stage to ask the promoters for money.

In the summer of 2005, I was asked to do a corporate gig. Instead of performing in a club, you perform for a company at a function or a party. And that's when I got my first paycheck. I was so proud. Then I was asked to do one show after another. Getting paid was so much more fun than paying. On the other hand, everyone expected more. The people wanted funnier jokes, the clubs wanted more people in the seats. If you can fill the seats most clubs will hire you. I could get at least 100 people to come see me, but not all on the same day.

I began to find funny in everything. I would carry a pad with me and write down things I thought I could use. Such as, one day in Vegas I heard the funniest thing I had ever heard and now use it in my routine. A man was arguing with the cocktail waitress, he wanted to get his wife another drink. The cocktail waitress said she had the right to refuse anyone. The wife stood up to calm her husband down. When she stood sideways it was obvious she was at least eight months pregnant. I said, "How could you let your wife drink, don't you care about your child?" The man stood back pointed to his wife's belly and exclaimed, "Oh! Dis'in aint mine." I asked the guy sitting next to me if I could borrow his pen. I had to write that down. I swear fact is so much funnier than fiction.

It was not long after that Vegas trip that I realized I needed more help to fine-tune my comedy. So I got a comedy coach, someone to help me go through all my stuff and determine what was really funny and what was holding me back; what works with an audience, and what doesn't. I found the best guy, Neil Leiberman, "The Comedy Coach," right here in the Bay Area. Sure, I had to schlep myself up to San Francisco once a week, but it was worth every mile and every penny. Neil helped me concentrate on the funny. He helped me hone my skills so well that I was actually getting calls to perform comedy from people I didn't know.

I was making it to the finals of every comedy contest I entered.

Then a friend I did comedy with, Bob, asked me to play his mother in a movie he and a friend wrote. His mother? He was like twenty-five. I thought about it for a second, then realized, SHIT, I really could be his mother. So I did the part for his movie, what fun that was, but now I know what goes into making a movie. WOW, hats off to actors! The movie is still in production, no date for release yet.

In early 2007, I was at Tommy T's Comedy Club in Pleasanton, California, when a man named Jeff Mosley showed up. He had a camera and asked all the performers that night to sign a waiver because he was making a documentary called

Comedy Ain't for the Money (see, I'm not the only one who feels this way) and he might use us. We all signed, thinking, "Wow, a movie!" But none of us ever thought we would actually be in it. Surprise! I was not only in the movie, I was featured!

I began performing once a week, sometimes even two or three times. And I was getting paid. Sure, I had a few medical setbacks, but I kept plugging away. Jodi Engle from *San Jose Magazine* did a wonderful eight-page article titled "Funny Gal" about me, which won first prize in the Global Press Awards. Then Marianne L. Hamilton of the *Saratoga News* did a story titled "Funny Lady," which won first place at the San Francisco Peninsula Press Club Awards. I had more than sixty-thousand hits on my website from those two stories alone.

People wanted to be added to my mailing list. I was actually drawing a crowd. It felt great. I felt great. I knew I was doing what I should be doing. Comedy has been a blessing in so many ways, and it's all about me in a good way for a change. Here's why I love comedy in my life:

1. I no longer need psychotherapy. After being in comedy for a while, I now know I'm normal. In fact, I'm probably the most normal in the bunch.

2. I can keep my children in line by threatening to imitate them on stage.

3. My husband will never give me another "gift" with an electric cord attached to it. Again! Ever!

4. People have stopped saying stupid things around me, i.e. "Dis'in aint mine!"

5. I get to laugh all the time, which keeps me healthy.

Laughter is definitely the best medicine! I know!

But the laughter began to die down when I stopped being able to drive at night. Which means I'm not able to perform as much as I want. For a while, I was lucky to get someone to take me out once a week, she was a fellow comedian and friend, but when she had to take a break from performing, that meant I did too. Now I look forward to performing once or twice a month. I can bug someone for a ride at least once a month, if it is not my husband it is Judy and Vic (the Puzzle Brigade). At least it's made me write more. It gave me time to finish this book. Look—one more chapter and we're finished. Unless you're going to go on and read my journal!

Chapter 10
So, It Concludes

I had to quit smoking pot. First of all, it was getting quite expensive. Of course I didn't know at the time that my kids were stealing it from me and then selling it back. But I was also gaining weight and getting paranoid. I kept imagining these horrible, ugly-looking, little green gremlins running around everywhere, trying to get me to eat cookies. "Here, have a cookie." In front of the grocery store: "Here, eat a cookie." In front of the pet food store: "Want a cookie?" They even came to my front door. Sure, you may not see them as little green gremlins; you probably see them as the Girl Scouts of America.

This whole "book" thing began as a plea from others who had found out about me on the web. People who were, by the way, just like me, out searching the Internet for answers. Could I now *be* one of those answers? They all told me that they had already seen a specialist and weren't satisfied with "We just don't know." They had already read my website in their search to fix themselves, and wanted to know more. In fact, they wanted to know everything. So I did it, I wrote a book, and told the truth. Hope you have enjoyed it. And by writing this book I relived my experiences, over and over, and it's made me realize how lucky I really am.

Plus I got a whole new joke out of it all…A funny thing happened on the way to the press. The young girl who was helping me edit, Katelyn, found out that she had to have her wisdom teeth pulled. She told me she was surprised after reading my story that I had never had my wisdom teeth out. *Shit*, where's the list?

Wisdom teeth: 1974, San Jose.

So wisdom teeth would actually be #2, shoulder surgery is going to be #26…Eh; I'll fix it later.

Along with these people from the Internet, my friends and family all convinced me that others want to hear my story. I hope this book puts it all together. I hope you have learned from my mistakes and my life experiences, learned what's important. Again, without the whole lung puncture thing. I hope you have learned that when you're going through trauma, it's so important to have family and friends nearby. I truly believe that the only difference between illness and wellness is illness begins with an "I" and wellness begins with "We." Having support always helps.

It is also important to love yourself. Love the flawed mess that you are. If you don't like what you are, here's your second chance to go out there and find what makes you happy. Fix it if it's broken.

And whatever you do, don't forget to do what you love to do—today! Very few people go to their graves saying, "Yep, I did everything I wanted." Don't put off doing the things you've always wanted to do until it's too late. Make a bucket list. You never know. I don't know why I had to learn this lesson in the face of tragedy, but I did. I hate the fact that it took me so long to get it. I am just glad I did.

Seriously, if you're not happy, fix it. Because if you're not happy, how can you expect the people around you to be? Your number-one goal in life should be to make yourself happy. Nobody can do it for you. You are the only one who knows what you truly like, love, and want. And if you don't know, figure it out. Then go out and ask for it. But be careful what you ask for—you just might get it. Then, once you're happy, you can help those around you find their own happiness.

I do believe there is a God. Regardless of whether you find him in yourself or in a church, God is hope and love. I am filled with hope and love. But I'm no longer a real religious person. I didn't lose total faith, I'm just more of a spiritual being. The difference, you ask? As a man I met in rehab most eloquently put it, "Religious people are people who are afraid to go to hell. Spiritual people have already been there; we're just afraid of going back."

I believe in one rule: do unto others. Nobody has to drill that into me, nobody has to tell me that it's the right thing to do. I just *know* it's the right thing to do. I will treat you exactly how I want you to treat me. I live by that rule—always have and always will. In fact I read an article which stated a Harvard biologist proposed that people are born with a moral conscience wired into their neural circuits by evolution. Thank GOD for evolution! (That's a funny line.)

Before the stem cell transplant, I would have said that life sucks. And I would have been right. For me, in my state of mind, it did. I didn't have much to look forward to. Sure, I had my kids and a husband who loved me. But at that time, it wasn't enough. When you don't have your health, even loving someone is a struggle. The mark I felt I was leaving on the planet was a dark, eerie one.

I wanted to do something positive. I donated my time, and a few things, to help our troops in the Middle East through the Adopt-a-Chaplain program (www.adopt-a-chaplain.org). They do such great things, like sending gifts and items that the troops request, including Oreos and Slim Jims; the troops just want a part of home. I'm happy I had the opportunity to do what I did for them. I have also been a huge supporter of and volunteer for the Myelin Repair Foundation (www.myelinrepair.org). But this is a little self-serving. They're trying to learn how to re-grow myelin in damaged brains, such as mine. Godspeed, Scott! (Scott, the founder, is also afflicted with M.S.)

I remember wanting to leave my husband, so he wouldn't have to suffer through my M.S. with me. I actually gave him the perfect opportunity to get out. I didn't want to be a burden or be responsible for anyone else's pain. He didn't sign up for this MS. I am so happy that he didn't take me up on that offer. His words exactly, "In sickness and in health". He has been there for me every step of the way. He's helped me through everything. My rock.

I'm so glad that I was given this second chance to change my life. I'm not going to blow it. Not many people get the opportunity I have been given.

I can't tell you how many people have asked, "Would you do it all over again?" Meaning the stem cell transplant. Would I do it again? YES! Even with all the thyroid problems, going into menopause, the eyepatch. It was so worth it. I'm not in a wheelchair. Medication is taking care of my thyroid problem. I can deal with the patch on my eye and all the comments. With menopause, I toughed it out as long as possible and then went on hormones. These things are all pretty much fixed. But other than my transplant, no other treatment has even come close to fixing M.S. It was worth every penny, because it worked for me. I am walking unaided, and getting healthier every day.

Once I lost my mother, aunt and grandmother, I began to realize even more how precious life really is. I spent as much time with them as I could towards the end. I wanted to know: what kept them alive and going as long as they did? They all said the same thing: family and friends!

But family and friends can also make you sad, especially when you lose them. My poor grandmother not only outlived all of her friends, but she saw two of her children go before her. That just wasn't right. She was doing pretty well until my mother's death, and then a month later, my aunt died. After that it was hard to get my grandmother to smile. It was hard to smile myself. Her health went downhill from there. She died one year, and one day, after my aunt. I lost the three most important women in my life in one year, one month, and a day. It still hurts, and I miss them.

This has made me appreciate the relationships I still have.

I no longer found my in-laws intrusive. I was thrilled to see them. We actually helped them find a house just a few blocks away. The boys could ride their bikes to see them. I could help them when they needed it. They never had to make up excuses to be in the neighborhood. They lived in the neighborhood. And I liked it; we have fun with them. Because of them, we began having Sunday night dinners together, like we did when our kids were little. This was our way to keep tabs on his parents. Every Sunday. I think everybody should have Sunday night dinners. Get the whole family together. Talk.

Most people don't have Sunday night dinner because they are tired, or are in a race with other people's crises. *Coming around the turn is Sandi with "Mid-life Crisis." Following closely behind is "Crisis in the Economy," and nipping at the U.S.'s heels is "Middle East Crisis."* The more people I talk to about all my crises, the more I learn I'm not the only one. We all have our own shades of crisis. We all have our own shit. And shit does happen! It is what we do with that shit that matters.

So much bad stuff is going on all over the place. We're all scared. Nobody needs more shit. Everybody needs to stick together, show a little love, and trust. Slow down. Smell the roses. You know. That's why we have Sunday night dinners.

Do you ever look at yourself in the mirror with two fingers pointed to your temple? Thinking, "I just want to shoot myself"? Well, you are not alone. Sometimes the shit that's happened is overwhelming. Come over Sunday for dinner. Everybody is invited. Tell me your problems. Let's share tattoo stories. Sit down. We'll talk. The food is always GREAT!

The dinner table is a place for everyone to listen and be heard, understanding that we all have a say. *Really* listen. Someday, someone may have knowledge superior to yours. Every person I have ever met, throughout my entire life, has taught me something, whether they know it or not. From how to act in a crisis, to what not to pack in a backpack to go hiking in the fucking snow, all the way to…the planet's hands-down best teething ring for babies is frozen waffles! All things I learned while sitting around our dinner table.

I love setting the table; it's symbolic to me. This is the very same table my grandparents shared with their family and friends. It's where they had *their* Sunday night dinners. It's the same table my father sat at when he was young. How cool that he now sits at that same table with his grandchildren. I love it. Around this table have sat friends, family, chiefs of police, Oakland Raiders, top executives, and addicts of all kinds.

People ask why we have Sunday night dinners, and I wonder why they don't. I do it so my family will stay close, so they can always come home and sit down to a good meal and talk about anything. Every Sunday night, we have an open invitation to my in-laws, my dad and his wife, my kids (which includes my nephew), and their significant others (if they have one at the time). Everyone is invited, and they almost always show up.

We talk about anything and everything, and have come to a lot of realizations over that dinner table. Honesty is still the best policy. You have to tell people what you want. By the way, ladies, if you haven't figured it out by now, it's all about sex. That's all most men really want. A little food, and sex. I know. I've raised two boys, a nephew, and a husband. Sex is what it always has been about and always will be about. Sex is what makes the world go round. Sex. Go ahead, and say it out loud. Sex. It's the reason we're all here on this planet—to procreate, so that we'll survive as a species. It is an instinct, an animal instinct. It's the most powerful and natural thing for humans to do, yet so many of us are afraid to talk about it, think about it, or do it. Hello? I say celebrate your sexuality. Sex is a good thing, especially if you're doing it right. If it isn't good for you, fix it or let it go. You, or you and your partner must be compatible, especially in that area.

It's too bad we all have to pretend that we don't do

"it," because we all do, and hopefully a lot. It helps relieve stress. We should just be able to talk about it more openly. It can be so much fun. Throw a pleasure party. Find out what floats your boat. If you are so old-fashioned that you can't talk about "it" to your children, then just buy them condoms. Put them in a drawer, in their bathroom, where they'll find them. They'll get the hint and appreciate it. I know! I do it because I don't want my kids dying from some disease or getting some girl pregnant just because we couldn't talk about "it," or they couldn't afford condoms. I think condoms should be free.

Plus, if my kids made me a grandmother right now I would kill them. I am so not ready for grandchildren. I'm still waiting for the day I can do cartwheels naked down the hall. Waiting for the last one to go off to college. Hurry, honey. No pressure, but Mommy has a guy coming to measure your room for a widescreen.

Illness and death are such difficult things to deal with. People who haven't suffered with illness don't know how to deal with people who are ill. They don't know what to say, how to act, or what to do. So in most cases, when someone becomes very ill, their friends stop calling or just fade away. It's hard to call all the time and hear that your loved one is going through another trauma. No one wants to hear that. It's hard on everyone. I have learned firsthand. I have lost some great friends, who just sort of drifted away, and honestly, I don't blame them. If the tables were turned back, then I don't know how I would have acted. But I do know now!

It's the same with death. People don't know what to say, or how to act with a person who has just lost someone. Rather than to just be there, be quiet, and hold their hand, people have this urge to speak. They feel like they have to say something. Or they don't call at all. If only people could read each other's minds, they would understand that they don't have to say a word. Being there is enough, but if you brought a casserole that would be nice too. People dealing with death don't usually eat right. Their minds are elsewhere.

My experiences have also taught me a lot about the simple things in life. It's true what they say—eat dessert first. You never know what's going to happen. Also, appreciate what you have and who you are. What I have is a new chance at life. And what I am is funny, nice, and beautiful. Once I realized it, everyone around me realized it too. During this second chance at life, I am going for the gusto. I am pursuing my dreams. Doing the things I want to do, to the best of my abilities. And most of all I want to laugh!

With all the problems and surgeries I've had, I still feel lucky. I am still walking without the use of a cane. I don't even care that I walk with a slight limp. My guess is that not all the nerve damage will be repaired, or healing just might take some time. I don't shake the way I used to, have no tremors at all, and the aches and pains associated with my M.S. have diminished. I no longer have to smoke a joint or take a pill, or worse, stick a needle in my leg to just "maintain." Now I do it for fun (smoking the joint, that is).

Sure, I have to wear a patch over one eye, which is inconvenient. But I can see! I'm also in menopause, but wouldn't I have gone there anyways? I've had problems with my thyroid, but so did my grandmother. She had hers removed when she was twelve, and she lived until April of 2005, which made her ninety-two when she passed. So do I really need a thyroid? And do any other medical issues run in my family? These are things we will never know. But what we do know is that the stem cell transplant worked. If I had never done it, we wouldn't know about that either. I am just glad we do!

I'm sad that it took me forty years, a serious illness, and a miracle to realize that all I really wanted to do in life was love my family, make people laugh, and write a book. Loving my family and making people laugh—not so easy sometimes. I live for the "I love you's" and those times when the crowd roars so loud at something I said. That proud feeling is the same as when your kid shows you his report card with straight A's. My husband would always liken that feeling to golf. He would say, "It's that one good shot that makes me want to play again tomorrow." I too live for that one good shot in every aspect of my life.

But in my opinion, trust has disappeared in our society. Nobody wants to share anything anymore. I say, "Slow down and have Sunday night dinners." Talk about it. No matter what it is. Say what's wrong. Be honest. Honesty and trust go hand in hand. If you can't keep it out in the open, it must be broken. If it's broken, try and fix it. If it can't be fixed, get rid of it.

No more secrets. I think everyone should wear a special T-shirt once a month, let's say the first. So, on the first day of each month everyone wears a T-shirt listing his or her problems. Everything that is wrong. Just list the problems on the front of the shirt; some may have to be continued on the back. I think we need to do this just to let everyone know they are not the only ones going through crap. It's a way to get compassion or help, or to just get it off your chest. Getting it off your chest by writing it on your chest. There it is—the way to achieve happiness. I know once I see other people's T-shirts I'll be saying, "I have nothing to complain about."

As an adult, I finally get what my parents and their parents have been saying for years: "If I only knew what I know now when I was your age . . ." No matter what age you are, it applies. If you look at someone half your age, don't you think it would be awesome to tell him or her all the mistakes you made so that they wouldn't have to suffer the way you did? Even if you are twelve, any six-year-old could benefit from your mistakes.

The way I see it, our problem is that no one wants to share his or her personal problems. Once I told people that I had M.S., people I knew who also had M.S. came out of the woodwork to tell me they did too. But some wanted me to keep it a secret. How can people know what you're going through if you don't tell them? Communication is important! I told people and look what happened. Not that I wanted so many other people I grew up with to also have M.S., but it is a weird kind of comfort to find out I'm not the only one.

I learned some stuff from my parents, and then I got to be a lot smarter than them. Just like the younger generation is smarter than me now. I say thank God for evolution. With all this communication technology, it's a lot easier to access the shit we should know. I sure wish I had listened a little more closely when I was young. Most of us are only hoping our kids—and all the young kids out there—don't make the same mistakes we did. You need to listen! Learn how to communicate better. Bring back service! Where is my fluff?

Everything is too instant; we're raising children with a "got to have it now" mentality. My kids aren't ADD, they're overstimulated. Fast food, instant messaging, if it's not quick, fast-paced, at high speed, turbo or supersonic, it's too slow. I remember when my father wanted to compare us to someone he would look around the neighborhood and that was his basis. You were compared to dumb Eddie down the street. With the Internet our children are being compared to children all over the world. That's a lot of pressure. They need to be children.

People are living to be older, yet we're speeding them through childhood. When I was a child, people at the age of fifty were sure they were at least two-thirds of the way through their lives. Now, at the same age, we're only halfway through our lives. Living longer. Is this a blessing or a curse? You decide. Then do something about it. If it's broken, fix it; if it can't be fixed, let it go. I've decided to take care of my body. I now do Pilates three times a week. Thanks to Helen (my MS sister) who talked me and Rob into joining her, and Tammi and Cynthia, our instructors. I am back to having balance. Wow!

I even go so far as getting a massage once in a while. OK once a week, but who's counting. Thanks to APD Spa (A Perfect Day Spa) for making it affordable, and William the Yoda-like master of massage therapy who seems to magically find all the kinks, then gets them out. Like I said, it's all about me! If I'm doing well and am happy, then I can be there for those who need me. You know the alternative. I do! That was my hell, and I'm not going back.

Some say our kids will be living into their one hundred and twenties. Can you imagine? I can barely imagine myself at age seventy, and that's in about twenty years for me. Add on to that another fifty years. Wow, that is a long time. If I had known I was gonna live even this long (which has surprised the hell out of me), I would've taken better care of myself. I didn't know better. If I had known better, I would never have…(Fill in the blank.)

I want to know that my life might inspire just one reader of this book, and teach him or her something that is life-changing. Maybe that person is you.

My Photos

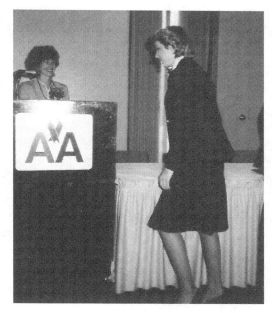

Me graduating from American Airlines flight attendant academy.

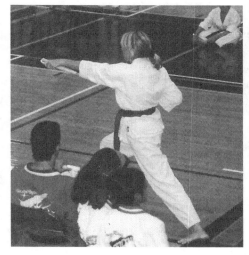

The day I won the gold metal for nunchucks.

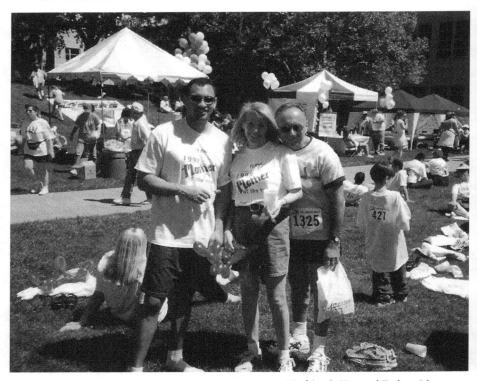

My friends Ken and Eteka with me at the MS walk when I was the *Mother of the Year.*

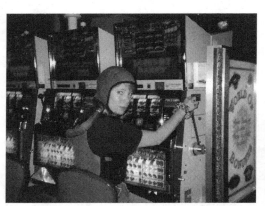

I would have tried anything to stop my M.S. including wearing a cool suit designed by Bill Elkins at NASA.

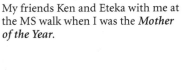

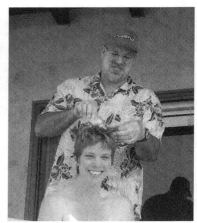

My husband dying my hair after my haircut.

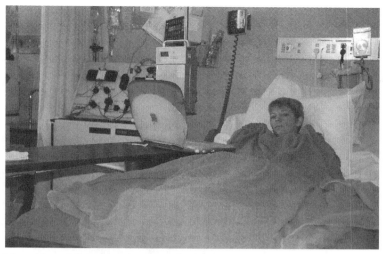

Me writing while I was going through Pheresis.

Rob finally shaved my head. And, see all the stuff hanging on the pole? Potassium!

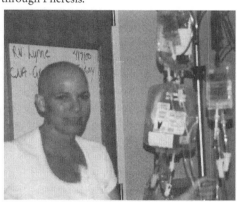

Three months after the transplant, I was scheduling soccer practice for my kids.

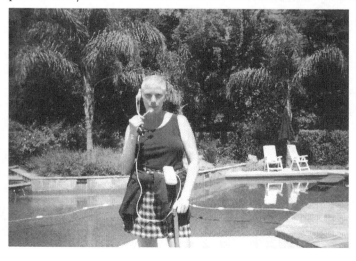

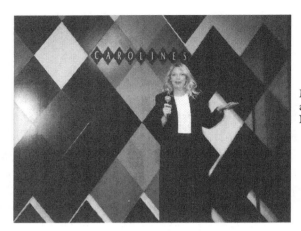

Me performing
at Carolines in
New York!

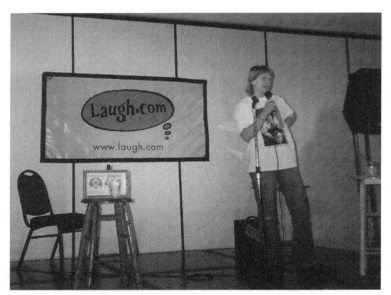

My first gig, doing an all night show with the late, Grace White, for a shot at
the Guinness Book of World Records. We did the time, someone screwed up
the paperwork, we never made it.

My Stem-Cell Transplant Journal

People want to know what I went through to get a stem cell transplant. I've told the story so many times, I've gotten sick of it. So I put up a website to help answer all the questions. But people wanted more details. So I went back and retrieved the daily emails that I had sent to my mom. See, every night, before bed, I wrote my mother a quick note telling her what I was doing, how I was doing, and what the doctors said. After the transplant I kept these emails for myself as a reminder to never forget what I went through. They chronicled everything I was dealing with at the time. So then I created a kind of journal from those emails that I could share with people who were thinking of going through a stem cell transplant. From that journal, my memory, assists from friends, calendars, and the magic of the Internet, I have spent the past few years writing my story. You are reading it now. Actually, you are done.

What follows isn't quite the original journal; I've left most of the filthy stuff out. But I hope this slightly modified version will help people who are following in my footsteps by showing them what I was going through, while I was going through it. It could be a reference point to help them get a better grasp of what they'll be going through and what's in store for them. So here it is.

January 7, 2000—Transplant 82 Days Away

Rob came home with the news that he had met a man whose wife had M.S., but was getting better by the day. She had had a stem cell transplant in November of 1999. I wanted to know more. Rob gave me her name and the name of the doctor. I called them both. First I called the woman, Deb Gafner. I wanted to hear her side of the story. From what she told me, she had been much worse off than me. We had some of the same symptoms, but we also each had our own separate ones. She convinced me that I should look into stem cell research. The whole thought of not having M.S. was so exciting. Next, I called the doctor to see if we could set up a meeting to find out more. My appointment was for January 21, 2000, at 3:00 p.m., in San Diego. I had to wait because Rob wanted to go with me, and that was the earliest he could get away. I spent the rest of the day looking up stem cell transplant on the web.

January 8, 2000—81 Days to Transplant

I spent five or six hours surfing the net looking for anything else I could find on stem cell transplants. The first time, nothing. I think I found about fifteen matches my second try. This was not a new treatment by far. It has been used for cancer patients for years and used for M.S. patients starting in 1998 in the United States, and since the '70s in Italy. I read about two cases from the U.S. So far, I had not found one thing wrong with this procedure. The way doctors knew it would work was because so many people who suffered from M.S. also had cancer. Of the people who had gone through this treatment for cancer, some had lost some of their symptoms and had not had an exacerbation since; some have had no new symptoms or exacerbations since the treatment, and a few said they were continuing in the same progression. I've only read about one person who has died. He was exposed to some form of spore from a plant that had been sent to him as a 'Get Well' bouquet.

NOTE TO SELF: Tell everyone: NO FLOWERS.

January 14, 2000—74 Days to Transplant

Dr. Mason's office called and told Rob that, while I was down seeing Dr. Mason, they would also like it if I saw their neurologist. They gave him a number, but when he called to set up an appointment, they told him that they weren't accepting new patients. So now we'd have to wait to clear it up on Monday.

January 17, 2000—71 Days to Transplant

Dr. Mason gave us the name of a new neurologist. I called him myself. They were going to rearrange it so I could see the doctor on the same day I was down there. They would call me the next day to confirm.

January 18, 2000—70 Days to Transplant

Dr. Sipes, the neurologist, called. I would be seeing him at 1:00 p.m. on Friday, right before I saw Dr. Mason. He seemed so nice. Not like any other neurologists I had met so far.

January 20, 2000—68 Days to Transplant

I had talked to everyone I knew who might be able to shed light on this subject for me. I called every doctor that I'd befriended on my horrible health path through life. Not one of these doctor friends said that it was a bad thing to get a transplant. Every one of them expressed relief when they heard that it was being done at Scripps. Nobody wants a back-alley stem cell transplant.

January 21, 2000—67 Days to Transplant

Flight 776 to San Diego, 9:50 in the morning. I hate flying; I always get sick when I fly! This flight was no different. 1 p.m.: appointment with Dr. Sipes. He confirmed that my disease indeed had gone from relapsing/remitting to progressive. I could almost hear my bubbles of denial bursting. He gave me my options. If I wanted to, I could go ahead with the stem cell transplant. Or I could wait. Or I could change my medication from Avonex to Copaxon, a different M.S. drug, and try that for six months to see if it would slow down my progression. I weighed it all out in my mind: Avonex, one shot a week, and be sick for at least twenty-four hours a week, and still having exacerbations and stay progressing; vs. Copaxon, one shot a day, possibly sick from the shot and possibly still have exacerbations, and still be progressing; vs. stem cell transplant (SCT), one to two months of feeling like

I do once a week, possibly getting better, possibly stopping the progression, and, at worst, having no change. It was simple. I HATE SHOTS. So options one and two are out.

3:00 p.m.: my appointment with Dr. Mason went well. I am their idea of the perfect candidate for SCT, because I wasn't too far gone yet. I'll know if I am a true candidate for this procedure as soon as their "list of tests" are completed. I'm worried about the oral. We were shooting for February 21 for the operation. The kids would be out of school that week, and they could come down and see that I was going to be all right. What could be more fun for them?

January 24, 2000—64 Days to Transplant
I returned home and called my regular doctor, Dr. Grellet, and told her what was going on. I told her to be expecting a list of tests from Dr. Mason and to call me when we could begin.

January 28, 2000—2 Months to Transplant
We finally had the list of tests that needed to be performed. 2 p.m.: arrived at Dr. Grellet's office. They drew eleven vials of blood. Once the lab work was done, Rob and I went to the hospital for the remainder of the tests. After all the paperwork was done, and I was properly checked in, they finished two other tests from the list, but informed me that I would have to return next Tuesday for my echocardiogram and pulmonary tests. Then they gave me a huge orange plastic bottle with a white cap. For the next twenty-four hours I had to pee into it. This was funny. The thing was about a foot and a half tall and not as big around as a gallon-size milk container. I left it in my bathroom for the next few days, eyeballing it. Hmmm, I thought, if only I had a funnel. I finally figured out how I was going to do it (I planned to be home day and night) and coincide my 24 hour pee in a milk jug with the appointments they'd already given me for next week. My M.S. flared up today. I was a little more shaky than usual, and I was exhausted. I think it was the stress from the doctor's office and the tests.

Tuesday, February 1, 2000—56 Days to Transplant

9:30 a.m.: I had to check in exactly as I had done five days earlier—same drill, sign here, and here, and here. Fill this out and wait in the waiting room. Then I dropped off my orange bottle at the lab. On my way to get an echocardiogram, I was called back to the lab to get a blood sample drawn to go along with the container of pee. Someone had forgotten to do it while I was there. Then I was finally off to get that echocardiogram. I thought about that scene in *The Wizard of Oz.* "Why do you want to see me?" "I'm here for an echo cardiogram, and my friend needs a new heart," etc. An echocardiogram is that reverberating sound you hear in a gym when someone lifts a bunch of weights and grunts. (That's pretty funny.) An echocardiagram. An echocardiogram is seriously kind of like the ultrasound test women have when they are pregnant, except now I was looking at my heart as it was beating. It was pretty cool. Then it was off to test my lungs. I couldn't wait to see what my lungs were doing. They needed to do a pulmonary function test to make sure the M.S. hadn't put any restrictions on my breathing. This was a breeze, but made me a little tired. Then I was done. Hurray! I called Raeina, Dr. Mason's assistant at Scripps, and she sounded as excited as I did. As soon as they received the results, they would set an actual date. They were now looking at the last week in February. This would be even better. We could go down as a family and spend time together before I went through this ordeal.

February 2, 2000—55 Days to Transplant

We had to redo a part of the pulmonary test. The doctor reading it thought that there might be a leak in the machine. It would only take ten to fifteen minutes. I fit it in my schedule that afternoon.

February 4, 2000—53 Days to Transplant

The coordinator from Scripps, Shirley, called to inform me that not all the tests had come in yet, but that so far, they didn't see a problem. We were no longer shooting for late February. It now looked like March 6th. I should go ahead and take my Avonex for the week but I needed to be off it for four weeks prior to my transplant. This would be my last shot.

NOTE TO SELF: Do cartwheels after the transplant.

February 7, 2000—50 Days to Transplant

My doctor's office called me to let me know that they needed one more vial of blood. Those greedy bastards. It seems that they did one AIDS test, but not another. I couldn't do it until Wednesday.

February 9, 2000—48 Days to Transplant

Done. The last test. Finished. All I have to do now is wait.

February 11, 2000—46 Days to Transplant

Dr. Mason himself called. There was a snag. What, did I have AIDS? Hepatitis? Was it my heart? Liver? Kidneys? I wasn't going to have this done at all, was I? Every single one of these thoughts went through my head as he went on to explain that there was a special machine that was used to separate the stem cells from the blood, a pheresis machine. This machine needed to be serviced, but it couldn't be done because the company was being acquired. Seriously, the pheresis company was being acquired by another company and in the midst of this nobody had the wherewithal to figure out who was in control of the service department. Dr. Mason went on to tell me that I should continue with my shots until I hear from him. Once they have the machine going, I will stop taking my shots, and then four weeks later, I could begin the whole process to getting my stem cell transplant. I told him that I really didn't want to take my shots anymore anyways. I would wait, take my chances, and the first available time, I would be there.

February 14, 2000—43 Days to Transplant

If I'm going to do this, I'm going to be leaving in less than a month. I need to spend time with my boys.

February 16, 2000—41 Days to Transplant

I woke up at 4:00 a.m. I was really excited. Our plane to Disneyland was taking off at 10:45 a.m. It was a fairly small plane with big ears. I decided to do something fun with them alone. One last chance to spend time with my boys, if something went wrong. We arrived in L.A. on time, and then the boys and I took the bus to the hotel. The plane ride made me feel a little off, the bus ride made me sick. I gave each boy a walkie-talkie, and while I settled in to the room (recovered), they ran down to the pool to check it out. My oldest son, Jim, came running back to the room and informed me that one of his friends was down by the pool, they were there with some other friends from school. I couldn't believe it. I had just seen this kid's mother, Laurie, the other day. She hadn't told me they were going to be at Disneyland. What operation was *she* going to have? I left a message on their hotel phone. When she called back, we made a date to meet the next day at the park for lunch. The boys and I hung around the hotel, watching movies and having pizza. We had fun.

February 17, 2000—40 Days to Transplant

I had breakfast delivered. After getting into the park, we rented a wheelchair. There was no way I would be able to walk for any length of time. So Jim pushed me. It took a while, and a few near-death experiences, for him to get the hang of it, but he finally did. We decided to go on several rides before we met the Coles for lunch. I could handle the rides where I could see what was going on in front of me, but when I went on Space Mountain, I thought I was going to die. I decided that this was my last ride. When I got off, I threw up all over my son Jim in front of the five hundred or so people in line. The boys were great. They pushed me over to where we were going to meet the Coles. Jim stayed near the plants in case I had to throw up again. Laurie was so sweet. She took one look at me and offered to take me back to the hotel. I kept insisting that I would be all right. She took the boys on the Pirates of the Caribbean, hoping that I'd feel better by the time they came off, and then we would all go for lunch. But I was worse. Jim took over and told the Coles we'd talk to them later. He took me back to our room and put me in bed. They took their walkie-talkies and went out to lunch by themselves. They kept in constant contact with me. They played by the pool and stayed together. They would beep me on the walkie-talkie, and I would stand on the balcony and wave to them. It was sweet. We went to bed early. Tomorrow would be better.

February 18, 2000 —39 Days to Transplant

We all three slept in. We had made plans to meet the Coles and their friends at Belle's Terrace at 10:00 a.m. But we had to get a wheelchair first. I did the smartest thing (besides vowing to not go on any more rides): I rented a motorized wheelchair. Brunch was fun, but the only thing that sounded good was fruit. We all ate and then began our tour of the park. We stumbled back to our room a little after 1:00 p.m. to get our swimsuits on and go by the pool to cool down and re-energize so that we could go back to the park for dinner and watch the parade, fireworks, and Tinker Bell. I think that we three mothers were more excited than all the children. We were back at the hotel about 10:30 p.m., and we giggled our way to sleep at about midnight.

February 19, 2000—38 Days to Transplant

We ended up getting on the bus to go to the airport at 3:00 p.m. We were on the plane at 5:15 p.m., and home at almost 7:30 p.m. I was exhausted. We all were. Unfortunately, the trip took its toll on me. I wasn't feeling well at all. I was running a fever, shaking, and feeling just plain exhausted.

February 22, 2000—37 Days to Transplant

Raeina from Scripps called and said everything looked good. They sent us a tentative schedule and told me the process would all begin on the 10th of March.

February 23, 2000—36 Days to Transplant

Both boys had their teeth checked out today by the orthodontist. Tom has to come back in a month and get his braces off. It's going to be so strange, for me to miss something that important. It made me very sad and depressed. I made his appointments. Now all Rob has to do is take him.

February 24, 2000—35 Days to Transplant

I taught my last art class today and had my last piano lesson until May. It was an all-around sad day for me. It made me anxious, and some of my symptoms began to flare up. Towards the evening, I became very shaky and more depressed than I had been in a long time.

February 25, 2000—34 Days to Transplant

Rob decided to make plans to go down to San Diego and look for a place for me to live. He was going to take Jim with him. They would leave tomorrow.

February 26, 2000—33 Days to Transplant

They spent all day looking and only found one possibility. Rob said it was kind of cute, and in a quiet neighborhood, but it still had a tenant.

February 28, 2000—32 Days to Transplant

The first thing I did this morning was to talk with Maureen, the rental house's owner. She told me that if we wanted it, we could have it on March 16th. The current tenant would be out, and Maureen would have the place cleaned. At least now I knew I had a place to live for the next two months. I had a luncheon, where all my friends showed up to give me their support. I wanted everyone to know what I was going to be going through, not for me, but because I wanted eyes planted on my kids at their schools and at their friends' houses. I wanted to know my kids were being watched.

February 29, 2000—1 Month to Transplant

Raiena faxed over my latest schedule. She says that everything is going according to plan. I'll have my first visit with Dr. Mason on the 10th. Then she told me the chemo date was moved up, so everything else will follow. Today was the day I began to feel really scared. Gayle, my best friend, helped by telling me about the birthday celebration next Friday that they'd planned for me at our friends' house. Perfect. For my birthday, poker at the Foxes'. If I win big, I can pay for my operation, or at least a couple of aspirin.

March 1, 2000—30 Days to Transplant

I went shopping. I bought Easter baskets, and Easter eggs to fill with candy, so that the Easter Bunny could hide them Easter Sunday. Okay, so I believe in the Easter Bunny. So what? I have done this ever since my oldest was a year old. Since I won't be here, I hope Rob doesn't forget. While I was at the store, I also bought a ten-pack of comedy tapes. This should be fun to listen to while I am sick.

March 2, 2000—29 Days to Transplant

I feel like I've talked to everyone I want to talk to before I go, except Shelley Newberry. I would like to see her one more time before I go. Not before I "GO," but before I leave for the hospital. She always has a calming effect on me. The Rohners and the Foxes (less Katelyn, their daughter, who is home with pneumonia) are now coming over here tomorrow night for poker. I do not need to be exposed to pneumonia right now.

March 3, 2000—28 Days to Transplant

Gayle called again. Both her husband, Ron, and their son Kyle have come down with a cold. It will just be she and Andy, her other son, along with Keith and Pam Fox for dinner. It was nice. Pam brought the dinner, and Gayle brought the cake. But I know the nerves are setting in. I was sick to my stomach again tonight.

March 5, 2000—26 Days to Transplant

I took the boys to play arcade games at Nickel City today. I began getting shaky and tonight I was sick to my stomach again. I know it's nerves. It might also have been from spending the whole day in an arcade.

March 6, 2000—25 Days to Transplant

Rob had a "work" breakfast. So he took the boys to school on his way. I couldn't sleep again. My stomach feels like someone punched me. Hard. I think I am going through pre-perfect life paranoia. Fear of having a life where I would not feel horrible all the time. What was I going to complain about then? I really am scared, and I really can't pinpoint an exact reason. The whole thing seems pretty daunting. I even sent myself an e-mail telling me how great this is going to be. But in the back of my mind, this old saying keeps going round and round in my head: "Be careful what you wish for, you just might get it." What did they mean by that?

March 7, 2000—24 Days to Transplant

I am beginning to get weepy. Every time I see someone, and they show any compassion, I cry. It's like watching *Oprah* twenty-four hours a day. Shelley and I went to Costco, and then to Chevy's for lunch. She makes me laugh; she always seems to say the right thing. I really am ready for this, and I think the boys are too. I can't believe I will be leaving in just two days. My M.S. symptoms flared up tonight. I may have overdone it today. I was running a 102 degree fever. Damn those chimichangas.

March 8, 2000—23 Days to Transplant

I am leaving tomorrow. I picked up my watch from Joe Escobar Diamonds, a store owned by my friend Stacey's family. Racey Stacey (that was my nick name for Stacey since we were young) wasn't there, but Don Edwards was. I hadn't seen him in such a long time. He was always like a second father to me while I was growing up. Don was my father's partner when they worked for the San Jose Police Department. Of course I cried. On my way to pick Tom up from school, I picked up Jim. Rob was home, so we all went to lunch together. I spent the rest of the day packing, but when it was time to go to bed, the tears began to flow. Tom was so sad. I ended up giving him one of my watches. I also gave him a journal so that he could write to me each day. As soon as I got him to sleep, Jim began. He wanted pictures. It was the most difficult night I've had in a long time. I'm going to miss them like crazy.

Thursday, March 9, 2000—22 Days to Transplant

Today I arrived in San Diego. It was a long, hot drive. The sun was beating down on me for most of the drive. Even though the air conditioner was on, it was still hot. My M.S. symptoms were at an all-time high. I was running a fever, shaking, and completely exhausted. We arrived in La Jolla, checked in to our hotel (the house won't be ready until the 16th), went out for dinner, and then to Vons for some supplies, and Blockbuster for movies. We watched *Eyes Wide Shut.* All I can say is WEIRD. Most likely because I slept through the part that might've given me a clue as to what was going on. We called my mom to check on the boys. They were asleep in their beds. I'm so glad she is there for them.

Friday, March 10, 2000—21 Days to Transplant

We woke up this morning and went out to play golf. On the grounds of the hotel, they have a short pitch and putt, nine-hole golf course. We played a few holes, but I didn't feel so great. Actually, I felt horrible. All my M.S. symptoms were flaring up. So we came back to the room and got ready to go to my first doctor's appointment. As we sat on the bed getting ready, I was shaking. I was sore and hot. Rob told me that this was why we were here. He was right. I realize that my life really has come down to the nitty-gritty, and I would like some of the fun back. Rob took me all over La Jolla, San Diego, and Southern California looking for a McDonald's. I was craving a hamburger and fries, and nothing else sounded good. I believe he drove for almost an hour looking for one. When we finally found one, he was so proud. I was so happy. At the hospital today, they took so much blood that the guy taking the blood joked about having to give me a transfusion afterwards. I saw Dr. Mason and Raeina. Tomorrow we start the whole process. I have to have a chest x-ray, more blood tests, and then it's chemo time. I am scared.

Saturday, March 11, 2000—20 Days to Transplant

This morning we went to the hospital and checked in, and it seemed like we were the only ones in the building. When we were introduced to the staff, they all smiled; they knew why we were there. They put me in a room right away. We sat there watching the TV, while a girl with cold hands, and cold sticky things, came in to do another cardiogram. I had to have an I.V. put in. Then it was off to do the x-ray. Then it all started. I was first given a bag of fluids and then a bag of Cytoxin, and then a bag to barf in. Cytoxin is the trade name for the drug cyclophosphamide, used to inhibit the growth of tumors and rapidly proliferating cells. What a horrible name for a drug, Cy-tox-in. Why didn't they just call it "Tumor-in." It took us until 5 p.m. today. On the way home, I threw up three times. Thank you, barf bag. Once back at home, I fell asleep. I woke up only a few times to drink a glass of water, throw up, and then I was asleep again. This was my first experience with chemotherapy.

Sunday, March 12, 2000—19 Days to Transplant

I woke up a few times this morning feeling sick. Rob tried to get me to eat *anything*. I was just not hungry. Just the smell of food makes me feel sick. I miss my boys. My temperature seemed warm, so Rob went to the store and bought a thermometer. I remember them saying at the hospital that anything over 100.8 degrees and I would have to call, or possibly go in. It was only 99.2; nothing to worry about. I slept all day long. Rob fixed the best dinner. It was a baked potato with broccoli and cheese. He also BBQ'd lambchops and chicken. I ate. We began watching movies again. We started with *Stigmata*. I had muscle spasms all the way through the movie, as did the star. The woman who we are renting the house from said it would be ready earlier if we wanted. YES, can we move in tomorrow?

Monday, March 13, 2000—18 Days to Transplant

First thing this morning, the woman called about the house. We can move in on the 15th. Today I started my Neupogen shots. Neupogen is the brand name for a filgrastim, which is a protein that stimulates the production of white blood cells. I will get one shot a day until they get enough stem cells collected. These shots are an awful lot like the other shots I used to take. They give the same feeling of being sick, like the flu. I pretty much laid low today and tried to sleep it off.

Tuesday, March 14, 2000—17 Days to Transplant

Rob bought me a bathing suit, so that we could go to a pool that doesn't exist. Yes, we were in the only hotel in La Jolla that did not have a pool. He had gone to get me some bras for sleeping and ended up buying me a swimsuit too. When he got back from the store, he decided to take me to the salon to get my hair cut. We had already decided that if my hair was shorter, when it fell out it might not be such a shock. Short hair is cool. Then Rob dyed it blonde for me. What a sweetie. The guy was cooking my dinner and dyeing my hair, and enjoying it. Either he is gay or something is really wrong with me and no one is talking. I did not feel good again after my Neupogen shot, so I went to bed early.

Wednesday, March 15, 2000—16 Days to Transplant

Today all I had to do was meet with doctors. Then we could move in to the house. We kept everything we needed with us in the car. They wanted to check me out one more time before they put my Mediport in tomorrow. A Mediport is a medical catheter implanted in the main artery under the clavicle; it's used to take blood and dispense medication. I met with the radiologist and had my pre-procedure MRI done. After that we moved in. It was a small cottage-size house, a little dark for my liking, but, it was better than staying in a hotel. Rob took me to Nordstrom's to buy me something for my birthday. Oh, that's right, today was my fortieth birthday. We had only been there for a short time, when I had this sudden urge to pee. The bathroom wasn't that far away, but no, I did not make it. I bought a couple of Kotex to soak up the mess. When I realized that my pee was orange, I sat on the toilet and my biggest fear was staring right back at me: blood. I quickly cleaned myself up and ran to tell Rob. He bought me the one outfit I had fallen in love with, but we knew that we had to go to the hospital. There they made me pee in a cup. And yes, I had an infection. With M.S., I was used to these. They gave me some antibiotics and sent me home. I was still on to have my Mediport implanted tomorrow.

Thursday, March 16, 2000—15 Days to Transplant

We arrived at the hospital at 1 p.m. Checked in, then were put in a room. They told us the wait may be longer than we had anticipated and that I should just rest there until they called me. By 7 p.m. I was getting a little nervous. Finally the procedure began. At about 8 p.m. I was in recovery, feeling a little sore. I kept telling the nurse that there was something wrong. I couldn't take a full breath. The nurse chalked it up to me being nervous and gave me some Ativan. Ativan is a brand name for a tranquilizer used to treat anxiety, tension, and insomnia. It basically knocks you out! Even if you had pain, you wouldn't care. When I complained again, the nurse gave me more Ativan. (I learned to complain!) After the second shot, I didn't care that I couldn't breathe; she sent me home. All night I coughed, and coughed, and coughed to the point where my ribs began to ache. One time, I coughed so hard that I swear I passed out for a moment. I was scared. I propped all my pillows upright and began listening to my comedy tapes; I was afraid to fall asleep. I thought if I fell asleep, I could die. The first tape I listened to was Brian Regan, and I thought, If I'm going to die, I want to die laughing.

Friday, March 17, 2000—14 Days to Transplant

When we went back to the hospital, they took one look at me and took an x-ray, and saw that my left lung had collapsed. No biggie, more surgery. It really hurt. They fitted a tube called a Heimlich into my chest and the pain went right away. It was just awkward. I had to stay in the hospital overnight. They put me on heavy antibiotics; one of them made me flushed and itchy. I honestly thought I was going to scratch through my skin. Twice I got up to go to the restroom, and both times, I left a trail of pee from the bed to the toilet. There have been many times where I've lost control. But it seems like it happens all the time now. Rob told me that Jim was flying in for a visit tomorrow. Tom didn't want to go on the plane without an adult along, so Jim was coming alone.

NOTE TO SELF: Buy some Poise. Not poison, Poise adult diapers.

Saturday, March 18, 2000—3 Days to Transplant

Rob and Jim arrived at the hospital a little before 10:30 a.m. Jim had the sniffles. I couldn't even hug him, but it was awesome seeing his smiling face. We arrived back at the house by 11 a.m. Rob and Jim went to get something to eat. By the time they got back to the house, I was not doing so well. Fever, no fever, fever, hospital. Rob and Jim spent the night in the house, without me. I was in the hospital. I got to spend a whole ten to fifteen minutes with Jim while he was here.

Sunday, March 19, 2000—12 Days to Transplant

Jim and Rob stopped by before they had lunch, and then they were off to the airport. Jim was so sad, almost as sad as I was. We didn't get to spend any time together. After the airport, Rob picked me up and took me home. As soon as we got home, my fever spiked up to 100.5. I remembered that at 100.8 I have to go back in to the hospital. It dropped down after the Tylenol. But right before bed, it went up to 101.5. Rob called the hospital. They said to take more Tylenol. He said, "That's fine for me, but what about Sandi?" What a joker. Since I had to be in the hospital at 7:00 a.m. the next day anyway, and given the amount of antibiotics I was taking, they had no problem letting me stay at home.

Monday, March 20, 2000—11 Days to Transplant

Today I woke up feeling pretty good. Last night I slept really well for the first time in a long time. We had to be at the hospital early for more antibiotics and blood tests. This was the same antibiotic I had the other day which the nurse called "red man's" antibiotic, where I itched all over. I told the nurse about my reaction the first time I had taken it, and she gave me something to prevent it from happening again. 7:00 p.m., we came home, ate a wonderful dinner, and went down to the beach to watch the sunset. It was magnificent.

Tuesday, March 21, 2000—10 Days to Transplant

Bad night last night. Every time I fell asleep, I had a nightmare, which would wake me up again. I missed my boys so much. Sometimes I just lay there and cried. I couldn't find a clock in the house, so I dialed POP-CORN, but the service didn't work in San Diego. I began to listen to my comedy tapes. This time it was Richard Belzer. I remembered hearing him on the Howard Stern show. I laughed. I tossed and turned all night, but I laughed. When Rob and I arrived at the hospital this morning, the nurses, again all decked in green, hair back, masks on, drew their usual nine vials of blood and sent us off to eat our morning meal—kind of like a bed-and-breakfast in Transylvania. After breakfast, they hooked me up to a machine that pumped blood out of my body, through the Mediport, the one placed in my chest, and back in through another tube. Like a Slurpee maker, but this machine was spinning and separating my blood, trying to extract all my stem cells. The doctors said they needed several million. My stem cells were orange and quite beautiful, if I do say so myself. During the process, the lab found that I had low levels of potassium, which helps maintain normal blood pressure. So afterward, I was quickly moved to another room to be given potassium from bags hanging from a wire hanger through the tubes in my Mediport. We finally made it home at around 4:30. Rob had gone back to the house earlier to cook dinner. He smoked a chicken on his little Weber grill, and it tasted fantastic. Deb Gafner stopped by with her mother-in-law, Shirley, to drop off her old hats that she wore after she lost all her hair during her stem cell transplant. She told me to expect it. Now her hair is back and thicker than ever. For a woman who couldn't get out of bed six months ago, she's doing great.

Wednesday, March 22, 2000—9 Days to Transplant

I guess they didn't collect enough stem cells yesterday, so I sat at the pheresis machine for at least four hours again. In the afternoon, I was supposed to be mapped for radiation. That's when they told me they had collected more than eleven million stem cells, and I was done with pheresis. But mapping for radiation had to be postponed. There was an emergency. So they gave us an appointment for tomorrow at 11 a.m., and then my CAT scan was at 3 p.m. My mom called. She wasn't feeling well and had been to the doctor. I was nervous because Rob was leaving in a week. We planned on my mom coming down to take his place. I needed someone here, someone healthy. And I'd been planning on it being her.

Thursday, March 23, 2000—8 Days to Transplant

I woke up a little early. I was thinking about the boys and how much I miss them. It was a very difficult morning. We arrived at the hospital about 11 a.m. for my radiation mapping. No big deal. I just had to lay on a cold hard table, stark naked, and keep perfectly still for an hour and a half, which is exactly how I normally sleep, except for the cold hard table part. The people couldn't have been nicer, and they tried to put me at ease, but when your back goes into complete spasms, and both arms and legs are cold, and are either asleep or in spasms, it makes for a difficult time. They were tattooing me so it would be easier to line me up in the machines when we began radiation the following week. I asked for a little heart that said "Mom," but they weren't equipped for that. The nurse just poked me eight times, dropped in a little ink. instant tattoo. I got one on each arm, one each leg and four times in a line from my neck to just below my belly button, then I had to have the CAT scan. Tonight I had a lot of painful muscle spasms in my back and neck.

Friday, March 24, 2000—7 Days to Transplant

I woke up depressed. Chemo just scares the hell out of me, and on Monday, I get a big dose of it. I think my depression was topped off by the fact that Tom is getting his braces off today, and I missed it. I just sat and cried. Poor Rob just sat there and stared at me. Then he suggested that we go to the zoo. It was my last day before I couldn't be exposed to anything again for a very long time. He helped me cover up my Mediport, and I took my first shower in a long time. It felt great. Then we went to the zoo. What a blast. Rob rented a wheelchair and pushed me all over the place.

We saw the pandas. I had heard about the baby panda on the news, and I wanted to see it. Rob bought me some cotton candy (my favorite) and a corn dog (my second favorite). At least I was eating well, and we were all over the zoo. Rob got his workout, and I got to see the animals. After the zoo, we came home to watch movies and relax. I noticed that what was left of my hair was now all over the black leather couch. It's falling out by the handfuls.

Saturday, March 25, 2000—6 Days to Transplant

Today we spent the whole day watching movies and cuddling. At about 7 p.m., I started to feel real sick. I was running a fever of 100.8 degrees. Rob called the doctor who said to stay home and stay quiet, drink plenty of fluids, take Tylenol, and stay away from corn dogs for a while. I fell asleep at about 9 p.m. I wasn't feeling well at all.

Sunday, March 26, 2000—5 Days to Transplant

I woke up with almost no hair. I looked like a newborn baby. It was 5:30 a.m. I took my medication and fell back asleep. We woke up in time to go get ice cream for lunch before watching the PLAYERS championship. My mom called. She still doesn't sound good. She has an appointment with the doctor tomorrow morning. She thinks she might be better by next week. I am so scared that she won't be able to come. I called Amber, my best friend from high school. Maybe she could come help me for the week: it'll be the hardest one yet. I need someone here who can help me. I am scared. I also called Shelley and Gayle. Maybe one of them could come down until my mother is feeling better. The PLAYERS championship was called off due to rain. I can watch it while I'm having my chemo. Tom got his braces off Friday. He had my cousin KJ help him email me the picture. My head itched all day. So Rob shaved it completely. I look so strange. We had fun watching the LA Lakers beat Sacramento 90 to 89.

Monday, March 27, 2000—4 Days to Transplant

Chemo is nothing but sitting in a bed receiving a bag full of gunk. The really weird thing is that the nurses enter my room wearing hazmat gear. Okay, it's not quite hazmat, but they come in with rubber gloves up to their armpits, masks, and aprons, holding the chemo at an arm's distance. Then they injected it straight into my veins. It was not that comforting, them covered head to toe, me under a thin sheet. It was one of the most uncomfortable moments so far. The masks, the gloves, the idea of poisoning myself all became so real, kind of depressing. But I did listen to comedy to take my mind off what was happening. Today was Margaret Cho. I hate to say this, but I think I could be funnier than her. After the chemo, I had to have six pouches of potassium. I'm depleting it quickly. And to avoid germs, starting today, I have to wear a mask to and from the hospital. I looked like Michael Jackson, and I felt like Howard Hughes.

Tuesday, March 28, 2000—3 Days to Transplant

They call this my day of rest. They only had to pump me full of one large bag of IV solution and six more pouches of potassium. I was given a daily diary. I have to report everything: peeing, pooping (they say that might start again soon), what I eat, how much I drink, and pretty soon the medications I will need to take by the hour.

Wednesday, March 29. 2000—2 Days to Transplant

Today started at 6:30 a.m., with getting my blood checked. Then at 7:30 a.m., I had to go down to the basement for radiation. It doesn't hurt, but the process takes longer than my body can hold still. They had me flat on a metal table, naked, with beams of light all around. It looked like a bad Las Vegas magic act. It was very uncomfortable. I couldn't hold still, they are going to try again tomorrow.

Thursday, March 30, 2000—1 Day before Transplant

Today I started at 6:30 a.m. again. They checked my blood again. Then back down to the basement for my radiation again at 7:30 a.m. It's so hard on your muscles. I'm telling you, lying on that cold, hard table, even for a short time, is tough. With all the spasms going on in my body, lying still was not that easy. But I did it this time. Then it was back up for more fluids, blood, and potassium. It took more out of me today than yesterday. Tomorrow I get my stem cells back.

Friday, March 31, 2000—Day 1

Got my stem cells! Yeah!!! The nurses and doctor called it Ground Zero. It was weird. The stem cells were in a bag just like all the other fluids they had been giving me. They put them back into my body through my Mediport. I don't feel much different yet, except I did poop today. Rob bought me an ice cream and some goodies. I had been craving chocolate, he brought every kind of M&M in the gift store. I began to get tired at about 7 p.m. I took my medication and went to sleep. I woke up in the middle of the night, I had to poop. As soon as I flushed the toilet it began to back up and then overflowed. It was bound to happen. The toilet never worked that great since we got here. Rob got up and put me to bed while he cleaned up the mess. I fell right back to sleep.

Saturday, April 1, 2000—Day 2

8 a.m.: back to the hospital. Same old, same old. They drew blood and ordered me breakfast and lunch. I needed more potassium. Where on Earth is all the potassium going? While I received my potassium, I listened to two tapes—Richard Belzer and Jeff Wayne. This pack of tapes I bought at Costco has been a lifesaver. We talked to the nurse and found out what my medications are going to be for the next two weeks. There are so many different kinds that have to be taken at different times. (Deb Gafner gave us the single brightest idea of how to keep track. She went to the

Smart & Final store and bought little restaurant cups with lids on them. Restaurants use them for take-out sauces; I use them for meds. You put the medications in the cups and put the day and time on the lid with a marker. Brilliant! But it still is complicated because you have to remember to take them.) The doctor came in, in the middle of everything, to listen to my lungs, check my legs, look in my mouth for sores, and then he was off.

Sunday, April 2, 2000—Day 3

Gayle Rohner came in today. Mom is still sick, so Gayle and Shelley are going to be spending the next few weeks with me until Mom is better. The time in the hospital was not so bad this morning. The doctor was there early, did his checking, patted me on the head, and told me how much better I was than they thought I would be. I still felt yucky! Gayle and Rob played cards. I was too sleepy. When it was time for dinner, Rob cooked Glorioso (my favorite pasta dish), steaks, and corn. I went to bed very early. I felt sick all night with a stomachache, headache, and constant diarrhea. It kept me up all night.

Monday, April 3, 2000—Day 4

Today was the worst day of my life. I had diarrhea so bad, and threw up so much, that I ached from head to toe. I couldn't sleep, even with sleeping pills. So I listened to more comedy. Tonight it was John Pinette, Bobby Collins, and Pablo Francisco. The three got me through the night. My fever spiked to 100.9. We ended up back at the hospital at about 7 p.m., and after hours of changing medications, I was feeling better. I even took a bath at the hospital. It was relaxing. We didn't get home until 11:15 p.m. Gayle and I were exhausted. Poor Gayle, I don't think she knew what she was getting into.

Tuesday, April 4, 2000—Day 5

Today started out almost as bad as yesterday. The cramping and diarrhea were almost impossible to deal with. At the hospital, it was the usual. The doctor was a little late. Towards the end of the day, I was given a whole new protocol. They took me off all antibiotics by mouth and sent me home with two pumps that hooked up to my Mediport. One pump ran all by itself all the time, and the other pump had to be hooked up for an hour at 9 p.m. and run it until 10 p.m. It gave me antibiotics. I kept falling asleep while it was running. This afternoon, I met with Dr. Backas. She's the bone marrow transplant psychiatrist. She met with me for a half an hour. She put me back on antidepressants: Zoloft 50 mg. for the first week and 100 mg. after that. I must have cried the whole time she was there. Can't she see that I miss my boys? Until Dr. Backas arrived, Gayle and I had played cards all day. It was fun. But sometimes I was a little too tired to concentrate. That was why she kept beating me (once again, that's my story and I'm sticking to it).

Wednesday, April 5, 2000—Day 6

I had the best night's sleep in days and had a new attitude. I am getting better by the second. I can feel it. Today started out great. I have mastered the antibiotic pump. But I had them set it for 8 p.m. because by 9 p.m., I am sleeping. I still fight fatigue on an hourly basis, but I'm feeling stronger. We were out of the hospital by 2 p.m. It was great. Shelley is coming tonight, and Rob is coming back Saturday. The theory was that Gayle would pick Shelley up from the airport. Gayle will explain how to get to the hospital and the stores. Gayle will be leaving the next day at 2:30, possibly by cab. We played cards all day, right after the regular blood drive, flashlight probe, and lung evaluation.

Thursday, April 6, 2000—Day 7

I was back at the hospital this morning, as always. Shelley arrived safely yesterday. She, Gayle, and I played cards. I began itching. From the top of my head to the middle of my back, I have a rash that feels like it's burning my skin, twenty-four hours a day. My double vision is the worst it's ever been. I am so anxious and feel like I'm crawling out of my skin. I had to receive more blood, and of course potassium, which always meant more hours in the hospital. That, along with the antibiotics, made it a rough day. Dr. Mason came in to reassure me that nothing too wrong was going on. Sure, *he* didn't itch all over his neck, back, and shoulders.

Friday, April 7, 2000—Day 8

Today I was feeling better, even though I had no platelets. So my first bag at the hospital today was platelets. I began getting cramps, so they put me on hormones to ensure I wasn't about to start my period. With no platelets, I had no clotting, and they didn't want me to bleed to death. Gayle went home. I was going to miss her. She had no idea how appreciative I was that she was there for me. Shelley and I watched movies and played cards all afternoon. I ate dinner and slept.

Saturday, April 8, 2000—Day 9

Shelley and I had a tearful goodbye. I needed more platelets and a six-hour drip of…guess what? Potassium. I am learning to hate that word. While I waited for Rob, I listened to my last two comedy tapes: Dana Gould and the Comedy Store's 20th Birthday tapes. I love comedy. It makes me feel good to laugh. Rob arrived at noon. He showed up at the hospital with his friend Eric and his wife, Alicia (friends of ours from Saratoga); they were coming down for a meeting and happened to be on Rob's flight. I was pleasantly surprised. We came home, and Rob cooked porkchops. I am actually getting my appetite back. I just feel punk though. I ache all over 99 percent of the time. I am either too cold or too hot. We watched a movie, although I fell asleep in the last half hour.

Sunday, April 9, 2000—Day 10

I couldn't sleep all night. I had diarrhea again, and it's hard to sleep when you feel like crap. The Provera (not a pasta dish— it's the brand name for a progestin compound used to treat menstrual disorders) must be working since my cramps have subsided, and thank God there's no blood. I was only in the hospital until about 3:00 p.m., and I slept the whole time after the usual probes. When we returned to the house, we watched the end of the Masters. Well, Rob did, and I slept.

Monday, April 10, 2000—Day 11

No sleep again last night. Of course, when we got to the hospital, I needed six hours of drips, mostly potassium. This is getting monotonous. Then there was the wait for the doctor. All I ever do is sleep, eat, and take medications. This afternoon, my temperature began to rise. First 100.8, then 100.9, then 101.4. I was scared. The hospital told me to take some Darvocet, a painkiller which also has Tylenol in it. It took an hour, but my temperature was back down to 99.8.

Tuesday, April 11, 2000—Day 12

At this morning's meeting, all the doctors and nurses came in to report on my condition. After the doctors and nurses confirmed all my strange goings-on —the pain in my shoulder, high fever, and itching—they informed me that they were going to remove my Mediport tomorrow because they thought it was infected. I have an appointment at 11:00 a.m. that will probably make the pain in my shoulder and underarm stop. I'll still have to go in at 8 a.m. for blood tests and more antibiotics, and then wait for the surgeon to remove the Mediport. Then I'll be doing back-flips and cartwheels down the halls. That catheter really hinders gymnastics.

Wednesday, April 12, 2000—Day 13

Today, massive amounts of blood were drawn. Then I fell asleep waiting to get my Mediport out. At 1 p.m., we entered the doctor's office. I was scared to death. The doctor came in and introduced himself. As we shook hands, the only thing that came out of my mouth was "I'm scared to death," and then I started crying. I felt so stupid. The procedure didn't take very long. He had to numb up the area. Then he just pulled, and it was out. I thought I was going to pass out. We went home after that and watched movies. I, of course, fell asleep during the last half hour. Someday I'll sit down and watch the end of all the movies I missed. I know, don't tell me...ROSEBUD.

Thursday, April 13, 2000—Day 14

Hospital, 8 a.m. The first thing they did was put an I.V. in my hand. They needed blood, and I also needed some antibiotics. We were out of there by noon. All my counts were way up, so I didn't have to go back to the hospital until Monday. Rob stopped and picked up a green burrito from Taco Bell. This was my first fast food from the outside world since my procedure began. I had been dreaming about green burritos every time we passed Taco Bell on our way to the hospital, *every day!* It was heaven!

Friday, April 14, 2000—Day 15

Today was the first day I didn't have to go to the hospital. Thank you, green burrito. I sat around and watched morning talk shows. I was very emotional, and I started crying when I saw this little boy who was going to race "For A Cure," which is a fundraising race for M.S. But I cried even harder when I found out that Donny and Marie Osmond's brother had M.S. I wish more people knew about stem cell transplants. I did get up enough strength to go to Harry's Coffee House for breakfast. It still takes every bit of energy for me to walk from the car to anywhere. I had hash browns with salsa and guacamole. I was so excited because my mom came today to help me during my last two weeks here. I couldn't wait to see her. When she arrived, she looked like she was going to cry. Even though I'd told her I was bald and thin, she must've thought it wouldn't be as bad as it was. The truth was, I looked like death. I had no hair on my body, and I weighed about one hundred pounds. I looked like a soap opera starlet. We watched a movie and I went to bed early. Rob stayed up answering e-mail., filling my mother in on what to do. He was going back to see the boys tomorrow.

Saturday, April 15, 2000—Day 16

Rob got off all right. The rest of the day I felt yucky. I have no energy left. I itch all over, and every time I stand up, I pee. Turnes out it is a bladder infection. So I just stayed on the couch all day, only getting up to eat or pee. I have N0 energy to do anything else. Mom got lost going to the store to pick up a few things. She wanted to play a game called Quarters (also called Ten Thousand). After one game, and losing only $3, I was too tired to go on. I went to bed. It was 7:30 p.m.

Sunday, April 16, 2000—Day 17

More of the same. Only now I have a sore in my mouth that hurts when I talk, eat, or drink. I woke up this morning at 9:30 a.m. I wasn't hungry. Nothing sounds good except sitting on the couch. My bladder is still infected, and it burns to pee even one drop. It wasn't getting any better. And after my nineteenth visit to the toilet—each one excruciatingly painful—I was beginning to lose faith, doubting the whole transplant process. Maybe I would've been better off to wait until they had more people that it had worked on. Mom and I watched a couple of movies and then went to sleep.

Monday, April 17, 2000—Day 18

I couldn't sleep last night, so I listened to a couple of the comedy tapes over and over again. First thing this morning, I took all my medications and then threw them all up on the kitchen floor. I was at the hospital this morning at 8 a.m. They had to call the lab to draw my blood. Then I had to pee in a cup again. It took a while for the doctor to arrive. We finally left the hospital at 11:45 a.m. only to go back to my car and find a flat tire. It took AAA twenty-five minutes to get to us. I was exhausted and so was Mom. In the evening, I threw up again.

Tuesday, April 18, 2000—Day 19

Today, I woke up with diarrhea. Every bone, muscle, and joint in my body aches. I had no control over my bladder or bowels. I am getting so depressed. I am wearing diapers. I am bald. I feel like hell! But there *is* a God. We didn't have to go to the hospital today.

Wednesday, April 19, 2000—Day 20

I still had diarrhea as strong as it was yesterday, so I am still in diapers. We went to the hospital this morning. The doctor thinks I have a virus. I am on a whole new regimen of medications and should be feeling better soon. I don't have to be back to the hospital until Saturday the 22nd. After the hospital, we went to get the tire fixed, but we ended up having to buy a new one. $231 for one tire.

Thursday, April 20, 2000—Day 21

Today I had a really good day. I felt I could conquer the world. Mom and I hung around all day with me just feeling good! Wow!

Friday, April 21, 2000—Day 22

I woke up feeling so good that we went shopping. I picked out three new T-shirts. But the walking almost killed me. As good as I'm feeling, I forget how sick I've been.

Saturday, April 22, 2000—Day 23

Today I had a very short fuse. We were at the hospital early enough for them to draw my blood and have the results back within an hour. But we had to wait until the doctor arrived so that he could go over any changes. I was pissed when he finally showed up at 11:50 and gave me the same notes the nurses had already given me. I was angry for having to sit there for so long, wasting my time. I was feeling good, dammit, and I could be doing something other than just sitting around waiting.

Sunday, April 23, 2000—Day 24

Today was Easter. Mom gave me an Easter basket full of my favorite chocolate-covered coconut eggs. I felt bad that I didn't have anything for her. So we shared the eggs. I also felt sad because this was the first Easter I had ever missed with my boys. But Rob did it. He got the baskets out of the trunk of his car (where I hid them) and hid eggs all over the backyard. Tom, Jim, and my nephew, Garrett, didn't miss a thing. I was pretty sad all day, but happy to have my mom with me. And I was happy I was still feeling great.

Monday, April 24, 2000—Day 25

Today I have my appointment with Dr. Mason at 3:00 p.m. but I have to be there at about 1:30 p.m. to get lab papers and get my blood drawn. The plumbers wanted to come at the same time so the owner will be here to meet them. I'm still feeling good.

Tuesday, April 25, 2000—Day 26

I felt strong today. I felt good. I had to be at the hospital about 8:30 a.m. to get lab papers and get my blood drawn. Dr. Mason was there at 10:00 a.m. It is so nice to have my mom here.

Wednesday, April 26, 2000—Day 27

I woke up a little depressed today. All I wanted to do was lay in bed and cry. I listened to comedy all morning. Brian Regan kills me. It totally changed my mood. We didn't have to go to the hospital today. I am still feeling good.

Thursday, April 27, 2000—Day 28

First thing this morning, we went to the hospital. 8:30 a.m. with Dr. Mason and 9:30 a.m. with Dr. Sipes. No one can believe how well I'm doing. I still feel a little weak, though. Mom and I played Quarters this afternoon. She beat me again. All evening I listened to comedy. It sure makes me feel good. When a friend called to see what she could send me to get well—candy or flowers?—I told her a new comedy tape.

Friday, April 28, 2000—Day 29

Mom and I played Quarters again this morning. My appointment with Dr. Mason was this afternoon. This will be my last appointment before I go home. I can't wait to see the boys. I'm getting so excited that I can't sleep. All I want to do is play games and talk to my mom, *and* listen to comedy. Two more days.

Saturday, April 29, 2000—Day 30

Mom and I got up this morning and did our last bit of laundry and began to get things ready for the ride home. It's going to be a long trip. It's one more day till I see my boys. I can't wait. I bet they have changed. I was exhausted from working all morning, getting things ready to go. I slept like a baby this afternoon. I don't think I'll be able to sleep tonight.

Sunday, April 30, 2000—Day 31

I was right. I didn't sleep well last night. I was a little sick to my stomach. I was afraid to tell Mom because she might insist on taking me to the doctor, and all I wanted to do was get on the road.

Monday, May 1, 2000—Day 32

My God, my boys look great. It took a lot longer to get home than I thought it would because we got lost. It doesn't matter. It just feels so good to be home.

Days 33-61

For the next few weeks, I had no problems. I was progressively feeling stronger and stronger. I was still tired, but feeling better. *Definitely different.*

Tuesday, May 30, 2000—Day 62

Today was my one-month checkup. I flew down to San Diego with Rob, and we met with Dr. Mason and Dr. Sipes. They were both so happy to see that I was doing so well. I was feeling great. Still a little fatigued, but I'm feeling much better. I still have my M.S. symptoms, but I'm feeling different. I can't explain what it is, but it's *different.*

Thursday, June 1, 2000—Day 64
Today, my right arm swelled up to almost twice its size. Who am I, Popeye? There was a white spot, the size of a pencil eraser, that itched so much. I began to scratch it. When the spot opened up, it was completely covered in slime. It was a piece of pencil lead that came out of my arm. It was so gross, and it hurt like hell! Then I remembered—when I was in fifth grade, I was stabbed in the arm by a guy in my class. Now, time to go to the doctor. Antibiotics. That was so weird.

Days 65-73
It took about eight days for my arm to really stop hurting. I was running a small fever, but feeling okay otherwise.

Days 74-104
I was feeling so great. I knew my body was changing. I felt so happy and began doing more around the house.

Monday, July 10, 2000—Day 105
I flew down to San Diego today, alone, for my second appointment after the transplant. It was very tiring. But everyone was very excited to see me. I was getting stronger by the day. Dr. Mason was very impressed. Almost all my levels were coming back to normal. He said I could wait for two months to see him again.

Saturday, July 15, 2000—Day 110
Today my left knee began to swell. Who am I now, a sumo wrestler? It was just like my right arm. It was weird. Something was festering under the skin. It began to work its way to the surface. I scratched, and out it came. It was the tiniest piece of red lava rock covered in green goo. It was so gross. Then I remem-

bered. When I was young, I tried to jump over my neighbors' red lava rock in their front yard, without success, and ended up at home with a deep gouge in my knee and a Band-Aid across it.

Days 111-120
It took me a few days to stop aching in my knee. I started to feel like I was getting better when it all began again.

Friday, July 21, 2000—Day 121
Today my left eye began to swell. I knew the drill. Scratch until something came out. This one was a bit more sensitive. It hurt like hell too! But finally, after a few hours, a small, green, gooey thing popped out. It looked like dirt. Oh! Yeah! When I was three, I was hit in the eye with a rock. It could've been a bit of dirt festering in there. Also GROSS!

Days 122-135
It took longer for my eye to heal. I guess I should've stopped picking at it, but every time I looked in the mirror, I had to do something to the hole so close to my eye.

Days 136-184
I was feeling so good. I could tell that my shaking wasn't half as bad as it had been. I was no longer running fevers all day, and I stopped using my cane while I was in the house. I was totally on the way to recovery.

Friday, September 22, 2000—Day 185
I was back in San Diego today for my next visit with Dr. Mason. I had my six-month post-transplant MRI. I have no new lesions. Nothing has changed. My counts were all back to normal. I was feeling great. My hair was coming back in. I was still walking with a limp, but I was feeling so much different. My body was healing. The little things that used to bother me in the past were no longer bothering me. Flying was no longer such a strain. I was

different. I could tell. Dr. Mason said he would see me in three months.

Saturday, September 23, 2000—Day 186
I was feeling so good that I signed up to go back to coaching. I'd be coaching my son Jim's soccer team.

Days 187-236
In the almost two months following my last visit with Dr. Mason, I began to feel stronger and stronger. Getting out on the field was a blessing in so many ways. I was out in the fresh air, kicking the ball, and having fun with the boys. I was feeling alive and healthy. Useful.

Monday, November 13, 2000—Day 237
I got a call from Deb's husband that she was not well. In fact, she was in the hospital. I wasn't supposed to go down to see Dr. Mason for another couple of weeks, but I bumped up my appointment. I felt sad and helpless. I could tell by Deb's husband's voice that she wasn't well at all.

Tuesday, November 14, 2000—Day 238
When I saw Deb today, I could tell that she was very ill. I spent an hour just standing at the foot of her bed. She didn't even know I was there. My appointment with Dr. Mason went well, and he says that I'm doing great. He told me about Deb and how she had a rare blood disorder. He also told me that they had already checked, I did not have it. The good news is that I've lost some of the double vision. Until he did a few tests today, I hadn't even noticed. I was actually able to read a paper. I had no idea Amelia Earhart's plane was missing. It is so cool to see the progression.

Wednesday, November 15, 2000—Day 239
Dr. Mason called. Deb passed away. My heart broke. I cried

all day. I am also scared. What if that happens to me? I don't want to die. I'm not ready. All of a sudden I began to feel sick. I had stomach pains and a slight fever. I was so frightened.

Days 240-255

I spent these days in seclusion, except when I had to be on the soccer field. I was afraid of everything. Every ache or pain I had became so intense that I had myself convinced I was going to die.

Saturday, December 2, 2000—Day 256

Along with Robin, my assistant coach, we took our soccer team to the finals. We took second place in the league. Go Tigers! As soon as I got back to the house, I secluded myself again.

Days 257-293

I stayed in the house and felt sorry for myself for the first time since the transplant. I was convinced that what happened to Deb was going to happen to me, despite what the doctors said.

Tuesday, January 9, 2001—Day 294

I began the day by feeling sorry for myself again. I picked up a magazine at the store to help take my mind off things. I went home and read it. Then I realized I had read the whole thing. I had read the whole thing without glasses. I was getting better, a lot better. I hadn't noticed.

Wednesday, January 10, 2001—Day 295

Today I flew down to San Diego for my nine-month exam, even though it's closer to ten months. This was the earliest I could get down after the holidays, and the earliest both Dr. Mason and Dr. Sipes could see me together. I'm doing so much better. They both commented on the fact that I'm starting to gain back some weight. That was the first time I've ever felt good about *that* comment. I feel strong. Everything is coming along just as the doctors had planned. I knew that I was going to make it.

Thursday, January 11, 2001—Day 296

Today I began wanting to do everything again. I signed up to teach art again at the middle school. I took over the art docent program, setting up the office and supply room. There was a lot of work that needed to be done.

Friday, January 12, 2001—Day 297

Today I ended up in the emergency room. My right breast began to swell to twice its size. Normally, I would have loved that, but it began to hurt. I had red streaks going down my arm and into my chest. It turns out that my body was rejecting my right breast implant. It had to be removed today. The doctor wanted to remove both implants, but my insurance company said it would only pay for the one in question, so the left one remained.

Days 298-321

I dressed my scar and tried to hide the fact that my right breast was a B cup (if that), while the left one remained a double D. It was very painful—more painful than I had remembered when they were put in. Every time the wind blew, I would spin in circles.

Tuesday, February 6, 2001—Day 322

I knew the drill. Left breast. Hospital. Left breast implant removed. I wasn't so scared.

Days 323-350

I honestly have not felt this good in years. Something has changed. My body feels so different. Like it could relax. My left breast still ached for a while after the surgery, but I was feeling better. Maybe my body was done spitting out all the foreign objects. Maybe I was heading towards getting even better.

Wednesday, March 7, 2001   Day 351

I was in San Diego for my one-year checkup. Everything is

going great. The only new thing is that I'm having problems with my thyroid, but the doctors say that they can fix that with medication. No need to worry. They think that's why I've been tired lately. Other than that, I'm feeling so strong.

Days 352-358
I'm feeling so good. I love being back at the school teaching. I love doing things. Anything!

March 15, 2001—Day 359
My friends were stopping by today, so I got up and ran to the bathroom looking for my brush. That's right. I RAN. How cool is that?

April 2001—1 Year After the Transplant
This month I began stand-up comedy classes with the San Francisco Comedy College. I don't know if I'll continue. But I sure like to laugh. I am funny.

March 2002—2 Years After the Transplant
I have spent the year teaching art and doing comedy classes. I'm having fun and enjoying my life. This is my second chance at it, and I'm not going to blow it. I went back down to San Diego for my two-year checkup. Wow! I'm doing great. My tremors have completely stopped. I never thought I would see this day. My double vision is completely gone. My thyroid is no longer hypo; it's now gone hyper. My eyes are beginning to bug out of my head. I look so different. But my M.S. seems to be gone. My new endocrinologist has told me that she'll have me back to normal in no time.

March 2003—3 Years After the Transplant
Three-year checkup and MRI. Still no new lesions. No one can believe how well I'm doing. I can. What I can't believe is how well I do on flights. It's so strange. I used to get so sick flying; now,

I feel nothing. My body has changed so much. I love how different I feel.

Friday, November 14, 2003—3 Years, 7 Months
I had to have a small cyst on my face removed. It was nothing serious, and the doctor could remove it from inside my mouth through the cheek, leaving no scar. No scar.

November 2003 through June 2004
My thyroid was still out of control. Every time we would get it going in the right direction, it would take a different path. I was getting upset, but I had other problems I had to deal with.

Wednesday, June 9, 2004—4 Years, 3 Months
The M.S. Society called and told me that they wouldn't be using me in the Comedy Luncheon they had planned for the following week. The people working with the headliner, who I was opening for, said that comedy and M.S. didn't mix. I was out of the show.

I checked myself into rehab. I had to quit smoking pot. I was getting depressed and angry.

July 2004 through February 2005
I remained sober and concentrated on my comedy. I was performing everywhere, from New York to Los Angeles. I was performing three times a week. I was loving it.

Friday, February 11, 2004 —2 Months Shy of 5 Years

I was rushed to the hospital with horrible stomach pains. That evening I had my gallbladder removed. It was riddled with vasculitis, a thickening of the veins. I began to get scared, and that feeling of impending doom came over me again.

Tuesday, March 2-5, 2004—1 Month Shy of 5 Years
I was back working in New York.

April through November 2005
My thyroid was on a roller coaster. First, it was hypo, then hyper. It changed more times than Cher in a concert. I was still performing and sober. But my thyroid was not cooperating.

Wednesday, November 12, 2005—5 Years and 8 Months Later
I had my thyroid removed. Now I would have to be on medication for the rest of my life. The thing was, I didn't mind. I *have* a life, and that was all that mattered. The only thing I didn't like was that my eyes were bulging out of my head. I had gone in to full Graves' disease. The doctors at UCSF told me I'd eventually have to get them fixed.

November through January 2006
I took this time off to recuperate from my thyroid surgery. It turns out the doctor cut my vocal cords and I couldn't speak loud enough for anyone to hear me anyways, so I just stayed home and healed. It was hard not doing what I loved to do. Now I know how mimes feel.

Friday, February 24, 2006—Almost 6 Years Later
I began performing again. I have lost my rhythm and don't feel comfortable on stage right now. My thyroid levels are almost under control, but I don't like how my eyes look. I look like Marty Feldman on crack.

February through May 2006
Aside from my eyes, and now sinuses, I'm feeling great. It turns out that the material behind my eyes has swollen so much that it's cut off my sinuses. The doctors at UCSF also found that I have a deviated septum. My sinuses are completely infected. I've

been trying to perform, but I'm not getting as many gigs as I would've liked.

Thursday, May 11, 2006—6 Years, 1 Month, 12 Days Later
I had a combination eye decompression surgery for my Graves' disease and sinus and nose surgery. I was under for eight hours. When I finally woke up, I couldn't see anything. My eyes had crossed from the surgery. They took so much tissue from behind my eyes that there was too much room in my eye sockets, and my eyes simply crossed.

May through July 2006
I was unable to perform. I couldn't walk, let alone drive. My face looked like I'd been in a boxing match. My eyes were swollen and red—even more so than when I was smoking pot—and the rest of my face was yellow and puffy. Luckily, I looked worse than I felt. I have to wait until the swelling in my eyes goes down before the doctor can decide if surgery can fix what was now a lazy eye. I did, however, find a guy named Steve Peixotto who was putting together a book about lazy eye. I contacted him, and he took my picture for his book. I also talked to a woman at *San Jose Magazine*. She's interested in doing a story about me and all I've been through with my transplant.

Monday, July 9, 2006—6 Years, 3 Months, 9 Days Later
I met with Jodi Engle, the managing editor of *San Jose Magazine*. She's going to do a story about me in her magazine. She was so sweet and caring. I think she'll do a good job. We met for several hours today. She thinks the article will be out in October.

Friday, July 14, 2006—6 Years, 3 Months, 14 Days Later
I had surgery today to fix my lazy eye. When I woke up, I still couldn't see right. But it was better. The doctor gave me glasses to correct what was still wrong.

July through October 2006

My vision is horrible, but the glasses help. I've only been able to perform a few times in these months. I haven't had the energy, and I still don't feel right on stage. But I am still sober and still don't have any new M.S. symptoms. I also talked to Jodi Engle. The article isn't coming out in October, but maybe in the November issue. She still had questions for me. I can't wait to see it. She wouldn't tell me anything about it.

Wednesday, October 4, 2006—6 1/2 Years Later

Today I began working on my comedy again. I'm working with a comedy coach, Neil Leiberman. He's supposed to be really good. My eyes are still crossed, but I can't get ahold of the doctor at UCSF to get them fixed. She took some time off for a family emergency. The guy who's subbing for her doesn't want to attempt to do the surgery.

October through November 2006

Even though my eyes aren't lined up, I am having fun. I've been working with Neil the comedy coach. I'm writing and performing again. I had such a great set at Tommy T's. There was a guy there who was filming the comedians. He asked us all to sign a release in case he wanted to use us in a movie he was making. I signed.

I finally found out why I couldn't get an appointment with the doctor at UCSF. Turns out, she has moved over to Stanford Hospital. I called and made an appointment with her there.

Friday, December 1, 2006—6 Years, 8 Months, and 1 Day

I picked up the *San Jose Magazine* today. WOW! Jodi did an eight-page spread all about me. I sat and cried. It was the most wonderfully insightful article. I felt so honored. It's incredible. December 2006 issue, pages 124–131. I'll say it again: WOW.

December 2006 through March 2007

I have had people come out of the woodworks emailing me, calling me, and leaving me messages about the article. It really was special. I have also had more than 60,000 hits on my website, www.sandiselvi.com. People want to know everything.

Thursday, March 30, 2007—7 Years Later

Today I had my second surgery to fix my lazy eye. The doctor woke me up towards the end of the surgery to ask me if my double vision was still bad. It was. She then began to tug the two strings hanging out of my left eye and asked me if the double vision was gone. When I said "Yes," she put me back to sleep and tied the string, which was the suture. When I woke up the second time, my double vision was back, but not nearly as bad as it had been. I'll need a new pair of glasses.

March through April 2007

I recuperated. While recuperating, I wrote comedy. I'm still sober.

May through August 2007

I've adjusted to the glasses. No more double vision. I've been performing two to three times a week. I played Bob Brindley's mom in a movie he is producing. I'm having fun again, and life is great. I'm so happy that people are listening to what I've done and want to know more.

Monday, August 27, 2007—7 1/2 Years

Still no new symptoms, and I would say that I'm ninety percent better than I was seven and a half years ago. Life is good. I feel strong and am thrilled to be alive and able to make people laugh. I got an email from Jeff Mosley, the guy who was filming in Pleasanton at the beginning of the year. The premiere of his movie is September 12th in San Francisco. I am in it.

Wednesday, September 12, 2007— 7 1/2 Years + a Couple of Days

The movie, *Comedy Ain't for the Money*, was wonderful. I had such a blast at the premiere. This movie is going to go places.

September 2007 through October 2009

Finished writing my book!

Friday, October 23, 2009—Getting close to 10 years past SCT

At dinner tonight for Bonnie's (one of my MS sisters) birthday, the girls all asked how I was doing on my book. Helen, the same one I do Pilates with says, "You should call my friend Jennifer, she just had a book published." Someone else suggested I get an agent. I called Jennifer, she gave me the information to get a hold of her publisher.

Tuesday, November 23 2009—10th SCT Anniversary less than 6 mo. away

I signed a contract with Wyatt MacKenzie Publishing to publish my book and have it release on the anniversary of my stem cell transplant.

Wednesday, March 31, 2010—10th Anniversary of SCT

My book is released.

Tuesday, March 31, 2015—15th Anniversary of SCT

The second edition of my book is released, with the following addendum...

Chapter 11
Addendum

My brother used to call me a weenie. And he was right. Hell, I was afraid of spiders and needles. Spiders because they're creepy. And needles because ... oh no ... what just happened? Oh that's right, just thinking of needles makes me pass out.

Fifteen years ago I was stuck between a rock and a hard place, and did something I never thought I would have the courage to do. But when it came to taking care of myself, I had to do it. I chose the needle. People say that I'm brave for what I did. The fact is, I was scared out of my mind. I was absolutely petrified, and seriously had no idea what was in store. The fear of the unknown. Glad I didn't know!

In reality, you never know what you are capable of doing until your hand is forced. Mine was forced by something nobody could define. Nobody, including the specialists, knew what it truly was, and it was robbing me of time with my husband, children and friends. Multiple Sclerosis was slowly crippling me and turning me into someone I couldn't accept.

MS had to go.

The traditional ABC drugs weren't working for me. I was progressing rapidly and had almost given up hope when my husband stumbled across Stem Cell Research (usually it was me stumbling, thank God it was my husband this time). I still wonder every day where I would be if my husband had not sat next to that man: the only man in the United States whose wife, at that exact time they met, also had Multiple Sclerosis and just happened to be going through a stem cell transplant to stop her MS. I say stumbled because I don't know what else to call it. I don't believe in coincidence, and fate had dealt me some pretty shitty cards in the past, so it couldn't have been that.

I'm still trying to make sense of it all myself. I just thank my husband every day for stumbling into that seat. He was in the right place at the right time. If not fate, you could call it luck. Before that day, the only luck I had ever had, was bad. That day is the day things began to change.

After all was said and done, still sick as a dog, recovering from the punctured lung, weighing in at a whopping 98 pounds, looking like tits on a stick, I remember wondering, after all I had been through, was it worth it?

The answer is still YES! But I still miss the boobs.

My symptoms slowly began to disappear. Don't get me wrong, I still have MS, it just isn't the same as it was. My cold sensitivity began to wax, while my heat sensitivity began to wane; I have no more tremors, no more speech problems, no more double vision; I no longer need a cane to walk, but I still have THAT dreaded disease. Multiple Sclerosis just waits for me to become stressed or overly tired, then slips on like an old glove.

When stressed I can feel it starting first with my speech. My voice sounds cracked and old, the words won't come out right. Sometimes the words come out garbled and other times the words come out close to what I wanted to say, but not exactly right. People correct me when it happens; I usually play dumb, it's too hard to explain. When I go to say one thing and something totally different comes out of my mouth, I feel like I have no control and I get embarrassed.

Then after the speech problems, I can feel myself becoming more easily agitated by everything around me. Stupid things send me into a rage or depression. Then comes the limp, and that's when I know I'm in trouble.

I have realized that avoiding stress is necessary for my

survival. So I have put limitations on who and what I allow into my life. If for any reason you cause me too much stress, pain or discomfort, like the MS, you gotta go. I did not go through all this crap to have it come back just because you are an ass.

A lot of things had to go.

My eating habits had to change, too. It wasn't long after the transplant that I realized my stomach wasn't digesting food the way it used to. I spent more time in the bathroom … or running to the bathroom, than anything else. I was afraid to get on stage: what if I had an "issue"? (That's what we call diarrhea around my house; the D word just sounds too gross.)

I could just hear it now, "Her jokes were crap. Literally."

I had read about digestive problems after radiation. Radiation causes changes in the mucosa of your gut, and can cause changes in the collagen tissues and changes in the vascular channel. The articles I read describe and characterize injuries to the esophagus, stomach, small intestine and colon. All of which I had. I was afraid to eat. Because everything went straight through me.

My husband (and again my savior) came home from work with a pamphlet about gluten. He looked at me so lovingly and said, "This sounds like what you have been explaining to me." He heard me? Did he hear the part where I want to go to the Greek Islands, too? And I know I had been complaining a lot about the bathroom; he knew I had been spending way too much time in there, so he wanted to fix the situation.

A friend had already gone on the cleanse diet to see if she could stop the aches and pain from arthritis. After witnessing my friend go gluten-free, dairy-free and sugar-free, the results spoke for themselves. It was another no-brainer. I took everything out of my diet. No more pizza, no pasta, no cookies, no bread, no cheese—no ice cream? No way. But I thought I could try it for one week and see.

That was all it took. I'm convinced gluten was the root cause of my inflammation and so many other problems including weight. I no longer ache in my joints and the weight just fell off.

But my stomach kept aching, and I still had "issues" every once in a while. So, it was back to the doctors. An endoscopy and colonoscopy, in that order (I made sure of it. They use the same instrument.), and then several doctors later, they realized that I had sensitivities to many different foods.

I was stripped down to broccoli, chicken breasts, rice, and water (which I was told to drink at least 8 glasses a day). This is when I learned why water can be so important. Water is a cleanser; it keeps you hydrated, makes things move more smoothly and is essential for life.

After a few weeks I began to add things back slowly. I was supposed to add one thing a week starting with dairy. Within five minutes after drinking a glass of milk, I knew. Nope! Dairy and Gluten are both on the new list of things I need to avoid. There were too many "issues" when I ate them. I was so tired of running to the bathroom and sometimes not making it, that it was definitely time to make changes. I could tell already I was on the right path.

Next I added beans. No problem with garbanzo beans but almost all other beans gave me stomach pains. It was a long process to figure out all my sensitivities. So I decided to step things up. The next thing I added back was eggs and sugar. I realize NOW how stupid it was to add them both at the same time; I just loved them both and thought I could cheat. Cheating in any form is not good. It seriously made things worse. It took twice as long to figure out I couldn't eat either sugar or eggs.

"Issues" were happening every day. I put sugar back on the list of no-nos. But the "issues" kept arising, and the headaches that I used to suffer from, returned. So eggs went back on the avoid list. Eggs, seriously? Who doesn't love a great hardboiled egg? It was becoming a much easier task to tell people what I actually could eat. The list was so much shorter. After putting eggs back on the big list of "things to avoid," the "issue" went away. So I added back sugar slowly. When I ate too much sugar, "issues" arose. It was hard to accept, but I had to drastically change my eating habits, for good. It felt like I was being punished, but then I began feeling so "normal."

It was difficult at first to change everything I had known about food. Then I realized how much better I felt, and it has made it all worth it. I wish I had changed my diet years ago. I would have avoided so much panic, discomfort, embarrassment and weight. I lost over 40 pounds. I am now in clothing smaller than when I was in college. That makes it all seem palatable.

As soon as my book came out in 2010, I began getting emails from people all around the world. A woman named Hanna from Norway asked for a copy of my book to take to congress to see if they would help pay for her transplant. She has since had the transplant and is still fighting to make it an option for others. She wanted them to realize that it worked and that the cost savings would be astronomical for everyone in the future!

Stem cell transplants are being done in the US, Germany, Russia, China, and many other places. People are realizing that stem cell transplants for MS really work, and want to know how they can get it done. Why has it been kept such a secret? Honestly, I didn't know. I've been screaming for fifteen years.

To me, it's an economic no-brainer. The cost of my transplant was almost $100,000. The savings on Multiple Sclerosis drugs that weren't actually working for me, over the past 15 years, is way over $800,000, and that is including all the drugs for treating "symptoms" (that by the way didn't work either): for spasticity, nerve pain, fatigue, etc. Those drugs layered on top of the ABC drugs push the annual cost to over 80k per year! That's almost equal to the cost of a stem cell transplant. And, NONE of the current therapies stop disease progression, they only moderately alleviate exacerbations. The MS drug market is an $8 billion-strong industry. Do you think HSCT (Hematopioetic Stem Cell Transplants) will ever get FDA approval? Hmm?

I watched a lecture given by Dr. Marcia Angell, who used to be the editor-in-chief at the New England Journal of Medicine. The lecture was recorded a couple years ago. The problem is, nothing's changed. It is still happening. The lecture was called, "The truth about Drug Companies." One of the most important facts she shared, was how much more we in the United States pay for drugs, compared to almost everywhere else in the world. Her arguments were astounding. Pharmaceutical Manufacturers in the 2014 Fortune 500 averaged 21.4% net profit, approximately three times the average profitability of all the companies in the S&P 500. Those numbers speak for themselves. And more importantly, why don't the drug companies have to compare new drugs to old established ones, to see if they work better? Right now all they have to prove is that their new drug works better than a placebo, a sugar pill. That pisses me off. The amount spent on marketing to doctors and how it's done is ridiculous and we pay dearly for this. How can we in the United States continue to allow the drug companies to overcharge us by so much when we know all this?

Messages began pouring in from people all over who had the same type of transplant that I did. I understand this treatment is not for everyone and everyone recovers differently, similarly to the way Multiple Sclerosis affects us all differently. But I thought it was important to share with each other what was working. We were all comparing notes and sharing stories. It was nice to communicate with people who understood what I was going through.

Speaking of communication, Tiffany Lilly, Marc Coppins, Barb Yoder Coppins, Nicole Baer, Matt Newsome, Judi Lecoq, Lisa Vargas Curtis, and I began a page on Facebook. We call it "Stem Cell Warriors"; we named it that because we felt like warriors. We have grown to over 400. Most of the members have had transplants already, while a few are still trying to get into trials in Chicago with Dr. Burt, or are trying to get enough money to go out of the country and pay for it themselves. They must like their insurance companies. Saving them all that money. Right!

A man named George Goss contacted me. George had it done, too. He was also having great success and wanted to compare notes with me. When I saw his page on Facebook, specific to the type of transplant that we had both had, I realized that it made my Stem Cell Warriors page look like it was done by a two-year-old.

The kind of Stem Cell TRANSPLANT we had, a Hematopioetic Stem Cell TRANSPLANT, is NOT the same as the stem cell therapy, stem cell procedures, or stem cell injections that are bombarding the Internet (and not working). We used chemo because chemo is the way to beat autoimmune diseases. As George points out very clearly on his page, "No chemo, no cure."

There is information on his page to help in every aspect of your Hematopioetic Stem Cell Transplant if you choose to do it. He tells you where to go, who to talk to, what questions to ask and how to get help. He also has people tell their stories. It is comforting to know that there are others out there who are benefiting from their transplants. Again, proof that it works.

When people ask me for information my first response is, there is a guy so much smarter than I am, you should join his page and ask thousands of us at the same time. Literally over 5000 follow his page, people all wanting the answers. No matter who posts, George always answers. Hematopioetic Stem Cell Transplant - MS & Autoimmune Diseases. It is a long and hard name to pronounce but if you are looking for stem cell answers, it is the place to go.

So, my transplant worked, but the side effects from radiation sent me on a new path. The double vision I have now is from the surgery they did to combat my Graves' disease, a side effect from irradiating my thyroid.

Everybody wants to know about the eyepatch. "What happened?" "Why the patch?" Well here it is … ready? After they did that first surgery on my eyes to get rid of the Graves', I woke up with my left eye pointing at my nose. So they tried to straighten out the eye, by cutting the muscles away from where they had accidentally attached them to my eyeball. It gets worse, it happened twice. So, every time they cut the muscles in my eye, the muscles became shorter. After that, my eyes no longer worked together. Because the muscles are at such different lengths they can no longer follow the same path. My right eye sees everything straight in front of me, while my left eye sees everything up about a foot to the left and tilted about 20 degrees.

Since the surgeries, I have had double vision whenever I open my eyes. It never stops and never goes away. It is always there. After years of eye therapy I could focus and see a single object up to 10 feet away, but I would get headaches. Everything beyond that was double. Having double vision makes you feel seasick. It took a lot of getting used to. Honestly, it is still hard.

Now I can see up to 18 feet, but I still get the headaches if I have to focus for too long; "long" being longer than 20 minutes. It puts way too much stress on the muscles, then they spasm. And when the muscles spasm, it feels like the muscle is tearing. And I might add, the feeling of tearing is very painful. That is why I wear the patch. Not a fashion statement at all. Without the patch, driving for me is impossible, and so is playing golf; so I wear the patch often, and going between wearing the patch and not wearing the patch is difficult. It takes a few minutes of adjusting.

My double vision, my gait and ultimately my MS, have placed many limitations on me, but I fight to keep my life as normal as I can. And now I can do the things I want to do, just wearing a patch. The hardest thing about the patch was getting used to my new lack of depth perception and the blind spot that the patch caused.

You would think having a blind spot would make my golf game more difficult. But it has made my golf game better. I can't take my eye off the ball, so I will never over-swing again. If I take too big of a backswing, the ball goes into the blind spot. I would miss or top it, so I stopped turning as much. Golf game fixed. I'm playing at least once a week again. Wasn't able to play for years. And I might add, won my first tournament this year.

My husband semi "retired" last year, so we moved onto a golf course. Just like it says on page nine in the "Marriage Manual." Retire and move to a golf course. We try to get out as much as we can, and love the country club life. I joined the ladies 9-hole group. We call ourselves the Neuf Troup. The nicest and most accepting group of women I have run across in years.

Now that I'm back playing golf, I hardly even notice that the patch is there. The beauty of the fairways almost makes me forget. Unfortunately, the putting always makes me remember.

The patch is very helpful in many ways, but takes away my depth perception. When I am at home or know my terrain, I don't wear the patch at all. I just don't focus beyond 18 feet. If I go out, you must know how much I want to do it, because leaving my house is hard. Putting on the patch every day is a drag, but livable. Give and take has become a way of life for me. Sure I have to wear an eye patch, but at least I can see. And, seeing two of anything is way better than seeing none. And that was where I was headed before the first surgery.

It took a while, but as soon as I realized that the transplant was working, I decided to not waste my second chance at life. I started doing stand-up comedy; I swore while I was going through the transplant that if I lived, I was going to do comedy to make people laugh and feel as good as I did the night I had my lung punctured.

I began performing and loved every second I was on stage. I had read somewhere once that humor was a great way to communicate. So, I thought I could tell my story on stage and if I'm funny people will listen. Comedy was how I got through childhood and the transplant; I could totally use comedy to help me get the word out about stem cell research.

The sad thing is, people did not believe me. They thought it was all a joke. I don't blame them; I chose to try comedy. It was my path. But, my story wasn't being heard, except by a few. One of those few was Laura Good, a friend I had not seen since our high school reunion. She set me up to do a TED Talk. It was the most exciting and frightening thing I had done since the transplant, but I finally felt heard. Hundreds of people contacted me about my talk. People were so excited to hear that it was real. And it is.

Right after the TED talk, I had a sore throat that forced me to slow down. I still sneak a set in when I can, but my voice is too unpredictable. Turns out somewhere along the way my right vocal cord decided I was screaming too loud and no one was listening, so it quit working. I had a sore throat and could not talk, so I went to the doctor.

This specialist knew what he was doing. He was an ENT (ear, nose and throat) guy. He stuck a probe up my nose and kept feeding it in until I felt it in the back of my throat. I coughed. It was a camera on the end of a long bendable cord hooked up to a machine, with a TV screen attached. The cord seemed to go a long way in. Weirdest feeling ever when it began tickling the back of my throat. I was afraid to swallow, clear my throat or move. The cough was involuntary.

The ENT turned the screen around for me to see (didn't anyone tell him I faint?). On the screen were my vocal cords, surrounded by muscles on the left side, not so much on the right. The specialist asked me to say "eeeeeeeee" then asked me to do it again only in a higher pitch. Then he said, "This is amazing, look at this side moving all the way over here." He was right, my right vocal cord was not moving at all, and it and the muscles surrounding it were completely paralyzed. But the left side was moving all the way over to meet the right side. He said that was why I can still speak, and he sounded surprised that I could. He also said he had only seen this a few times. It was caused from either a severe blow to the head (yep I had that) or it could be from thyroid surgery (yep had that, too) and last it could be from a car accident (okay, which one was it – had 18 of those).

So I asked what do I do now? The specialist said, use your voice as little as possible, avoid stress, DO NOT expose yourself to illness ever, and especially avoid people with sore throats. Then he added that I had a nodule on my left vocal cord; if I ever get sick enough and cough too hard, I could lose my voice permanently. I walked out of that office so sad; all I could think about was would I be able to do comedy again?

The reality was, yes I could do comedy, just not as much as I had been doing over the past 14 years. I had to pick and choose. I had the best excuse to only do the shows I wanted to do.

When I told my friends what was going on, they asked if it hurts. It really doesn't hurt so much as it feels like I always have to clear my throat. And when I talk now, it feels like I am screaming at the top of my lungs just to speak at a normal level, and sometimes it only comes out a whisper. It is really hard to talk when there is any noise around, like in a restaurant. So I just don't go out or talk as much as I used to. My husband is thrilled (about the not talking so much part).

To this day, fifteen years later, I have no new lesions, no active lesions, and most of my symptoms are gone. The only things that make it act up are STRESS or getting overly tired.

What have I learned through all this? To be who you are. To take care of yourself first, so that you can take care of those around you. You alone choose your path. If you choose to invite chaos down your path, then chaos will follow.

When I was young I saw a lot of tragedy. Back then, I

thought that if you are not laughing, you are crying. I seriously didn't know you could just, "be." Personally, I just want to "be" happy. Still being married to the love of my life, and no longer suffering with Multiple Sclerosis on a daily basis, has gotten me there. I say thanks to my husband and my doctors at Scripps in San Diego for my Stem Cell Transplant. So happy it worked for me, and that others are finally finding out that it is working for them, too.

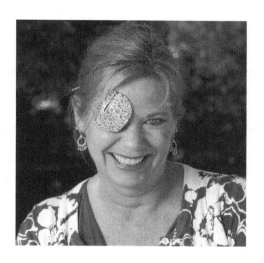

Sandi Selvi

Stem-Cell Transplant Recipient & Comedian

Sandi is available as a...

- M.S. Recovery Success Story Spokeswoman
- Stem-Cell Transplant Advocate
- Presenter
- Keynote Speaker
- Comic Entertainer

www.SandiSelvi.com

51096093R00107

Made in the USA
Lexington, KY
31 August 2019